Advance Praise for Spirit in Session

"A real gem! Remarkably accessible, this book makes the spiritual dimension of therapy come alive. Jones is a masterful educator and clinician who skillfully leads the reader through the meanings and methods of spiritually integrated psychotherapy. His wisdom, warmth, humor, openness, faithfulness, and humanity fairly radiate from each page. This book will be savored by newcomers and seasoned mental health providers alike regardless of their own religious and spiritual orientations."

—**Kenneth I. Pargament**, PhD, professor of psychology,
Bowling Green State University, author of *Spiritually Integrated
Psychotherapy: Understanding and Addressing the Sacred*

"Spirituality is one of the most important topics for most psychotherapy clients and yet it is one of the most awkward topics for therapists to bring up and discuss. In this beautifully written book, Russell Siler Jones offers practical advice to therapists on virtually every aspect of bringing spiritual discussions into their offices."

—**Richard C. Schwartz**, PhD, founding developer
of the Internal Family Systems model of psychotherapy

"This eminently readable, compelling, and inspiring book takes readers—heart, mind, and soul—into what actually happens in spiritually oriented therapy conversations. Russell Jones is a compassionate, committed, and elegantly simple mentor for therapists who want to help clients draw upon their spirituality in life-giving ways. *Spirit in Session* deserves to be a required textbook in every 'Intro to Therapy' course."

—**Carrie Doehring**, PhD, professor of pastoral care
and counseling, Iliff School of Theology, author of
The Practice of Pastoral Care: A Postmodern Approach

"*Spirit in Session* is an outstanding handbook for teaching. Russell Jones's exceptional mastery of both psychotherapy and spiritual inquiry guides therapists and their clients to discover spiritual encounters within the everydayness of routine psychotherapy sessions. Therapists may be surprised to learn that they need only their accustomed repertoire of interview skills, not a degree in theology or special techniques or religious-talk, in order to help clients find fresh meaning and new directions through spiritual inquiry."

—**James L. Griffith**, MD, Leon M. Yochelson Professor
and Chair, GWU School of Medicine and Health Sciences,
author *Religion that Heals, Religion that Harms*

"I had no time for another book endorsement so intended to say no, but then I opened the first page of Russell Siler Jones's book and couldn't stop reading. *Spirit in Session* is a creative, warm, clinically-relevant look at how spirituality can inform the life and work of a psychotherapist."

—**Mark R McMinn** PhD, professor and director of faith integration, Graduate School of Clinical Psychology, George Fox University, past president of APA's Society for the Psychology of Religion and Spirituality, author of *The Science of Virtue: Why Positive Psychology Matters to the Church*

"What makes *Spirit in Session* so distinctive and laudable is Jones's consideration of the therapist's own spirituality and spiritual countertransference, and how these can be ethically and effectively utilized in therapy. He does this in a conversational, relational, and humorous style that beginning and seasoned therapists alike will relish. This book also manages to be spiritually evocative without feeling prescriptive or heavy-handed. Reading it was like taking a psychospiritual retreat."

—**Rev. Jill L. Snodgrass**, PhD, associate professor, Department of Pastoral Counseling and Spiritual Care, Loyola College of Arts and Sciences, coeditor of *Understanding Pastoral Counseling*

"I loved reading Russell Jones' wonderful book, *Spirit in Session*. . . . I felt like I was having a conversation with a kind and wise friend who was sharing his experiences and wisdom in a warm and generous way. . . . I recommend the book for all psychotherapists, but especially those who wish to gain more insight into how to honor in sensitive and competent ways the resources of their clients' spirituality."

—**P. Scott Richards**, PhD, past president of APA's Society for the Psychology of Religion and Spirituality, coauthor of *A Spiritual Strategy for Counseling and Psychotherapy*

"If you've been yearning for some clues on how to ethically, responsibly, and effectively weave spirituality into your psychotherapeutic practice, consider this a trail guide and Russell Siler Jones as your traveling companion. Written in his erudite but down-to-earth voice, this book will help you feel more confident treading around this hot-button subject matter. . . . Furthermore, for anyone whose professional work involves addressing the spiritual needs of clients or patients—from board certified chaplains to other healthcare providers who wish to feel more confident in their conversations about meaning, purpose, and quality of life (in a word, spirituality)—this book is a great resource."

—**Rev. Amy Greene**, DMin, director of spiritual care, Cleveland Clinic

"Russell Siler Jones makes the enterprise of spiritual conversation in psychotherapy accessible. His approach is practical and yet illuminating, offering guidance for experienced clinicians as well as for clinicians who may just be dipping a toe into their clients' spirituality. And his voice is so warm, inviting, and encouraging that the reader will feel on much more solid ground engaging the spiritual lives of his or her clients."
—**Eileen M. Russell**, PhD, senior faculty,
AEDP Institute, author of *Restoring Resilience*

"[A] fresh, unique perspective on the process of ethically integrating clients' religion/spirituality into clinical practice . . . The rich case examples woven throughout help make this book relatable for mental and behavioral health practitioners at any level—whether you are just starting your journey as a therapist or have been in practice for decades. Similarly, whether you have always integrated clients' spirituality or are just beginning to explore this area of clients' lives more intentionally, you will find considerable wisdom within these pages."
—**Holly K. Oxhandler**, PhD, LMSW, assistant professor and
associate dean for research & faculty development, Baylor University

"Russell Siler Jones is a skilled clinician whose wisdom and understanding come through in this beautifully written, sensitive, and practical book. . . . This text is dynamic, thoughtful, and case-based in its multiple approaches to working with the spiritual experiences clients' and therapists have . . . [It] is a must read for all helping professionals."
—**Samuel T. Gladding**, PhD, professor of counseling, Wake Forest
University, author of *Counseling: A Comprehensive Profession*

"This book is a widely accessible and adaptable professional resource for understanding spirituality in therapeutic settings. It belongs on the shelves of pastoral care workers and therapists working with clients because, as the author reminds us, all people are spiritual."
—**Jennifer Ripley**, PhD, professor of psychology and
Hughes Endowed Chair, Regent University

"[An] excellent resource for clinicians to increase their comfort with—and competence in using—spirituality in clinical practice. Engaging and well-written, this brief book condenses the professional practice of incorporating spirituality in therapy, based on clinical experience, with a little research thrown in for good measure. . . . [C]ompelling and thought-provoking."
—**Kevin A. Harris**, PhD, LP, HSP, assistant professor
of psychology, Our Lady of the Lake University

SPIRIT IN SESSION

SPIRIT IN SESSION

Working with Your Client's Spirituality
(and Your Own) in Psychotherapy

Russell Siler Jones

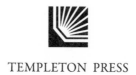

TEMPLETON PRESS

Templeton Press
300 Conshohocken State Road, Suite 500
West Conshohocken, PA 19428
www.templetonpress.org

Set in Minion by Pro Production Graphic Services

Library of Congress Control Number: 2019936421

ISBN: 978-1-59947-561-5 (pbk)

This paper meets the requirements of ANSI/NISO Z39.48-1992 (Permanence of Paper).

A catalogue record for this book is available from the Library of Congress.

19 20 21 22 23   10 9 8 7 6 5 4 3 2 1

Printed in the United States of America.

Can you love people and lead them
    without imposing your will?
                            —*Tao Te Ching*

Let me keep my distance, always, from those
    who think they have the answers.
Let me keep company always with those who say
"Look!" and laugh in astonishment,
    and bow their heads.
                    —*Mary Oliver, "Mysteries, Yes"*

Contents

PART ONE

Introduction

1

About This Book

I RECENTLY RAN INTO A THERAPIST FRIEND AT A CONFERENCE.

"Oh! Russell!" she said. "I was hoping you would be here. I want to talk with you about a client I'm working with."

"Let's hear it!"

"So, this client is in her mid-fifties, and she's sort of depressed. A lot of her friends have died in the past few years. A few more have terminal illnesses, and all these deaths and illnesses have made her think a lot about death.

"In the first few sessions she'd drop in these little bits of information about her spirituality. She grew up Catholic, but she doesn't go anymore. She watches a preacher online named Andy Stanley. I don't know who that is, but anyway."

"Anyway."

"Anyway, I didn't know what to say about all the spiritual stuff she'd drop in, but it didn't seem like it was the main thing. I'd just nod my head, say 'Uh-huh,' and then she'd be on to something else."

I nodded my head and said, "Uh-huh."

"Stop it."

"I'll try. Can't promise."

"Then in the last session, I realize: she's been dropping these spiritual hints to warm me up for what I now think is the main thing she's coming to therapy about. She said, 'Andy Stanley says we're never going to be really at peace until we're with God in heaven. But if that's the case, why not just let go of this life and move on to the next one? What's the reason for living now?'

"She's not suicidal. I checked that out. She's just not sure what the point of living is. And I didn't know what to say to her. I mean, I know what I think about that. But I didn't know what to say to her or even what questions to ask that wouldn't feel like I'm doubting her assumptions and being disrespectful. So I didn't say much of anything, really, and that didn't feel right either. You know what I mean?"

"I do. Definitely. The ways you'd respond to most any other topic—with curiosity, respect, 'Tell me more about that'—it's like you couldn't do that because the topic was religion."

"Right! This spiritual stuff is so personal, so intimate, so . . . core. I was worried that if I asked about it at all, it would sound like I was challenging it or being suspicious of it. So I sort of froze. But I think this is the main thing she's needing to talk about, and I need to find a way to go there with her.

"How do I do that?"

HOW DO I DO THAT?

"How do I do that?" is what the rest of this book is about.

I've been a therapist now for twenty-seven years, and I've needed answers to that question every step of the way. The people who've come to talk with me have always wanted more than just relief from symptoms of depression, anxiety, and the like. They want that too, but even more, they want help to live more satisfying and meaningful lives.[1] Sometimes they're asking explicit spiritual questions, such as, "What does God want me to do?" But more often, they're asking questions with an implicit spiritual subtext: "Who am I, really?" "What's going to make me happy?" "Is 'make me happy' even the point?" Again and again, people invite me into the most haunted and hallowed spaces of their lives, and again and again, I am blown away by the magnitude and meaning of what happens when we go there. It is such a privilege—and such a responsibility. "How do I do that?"

For most of these twenty-seven years, I've also been in conversation with other therapists about that question—sometimes by phone, sometimes at conferences, sometimes in supervision. Since 2008 I've been director of the Residency in Psychotherapy and Spirituality for CareNet (a statewide counseling network of Wake Forest Baptist Medical Center, in North Carolina), where I teach and supervise associate-licensed therapists in the first two to three years of their careers. I've also helped write a thirty-hour continuing education psychotherapy and spirituality curriculum for therapists.

One thing these teaching and supervising roles have taught me is this: most therapists aren't looking for lots of theory. They're looking for practical help: "What does a spiritual conversation sound like in therapy?" "How do I talk about this stuff in a down-to-earth way?" "How do I show respect for spirituality but not make such a big deal that the client and I end up feeling too nervous to have a decent conversation?" "What do I do when a client says something spiritually that I really disagree with?" "What do I actually say? And when do I say it?"

Spirituality, of course, does not shrink and fold itself tightly into the pages of a how-to manual. Spirituality is about mystery, meaning, and transformation. It occupies a realm of connection and knowing beyond the world of facts, formula, and efficiency. We can have guides in this realm, but no guide can prepare us for everything we will encounter.

It is the same with psychotherapy that engages spirituality. All therapists must find their own way, with each client, to work with spirituality. No book and no instructor can spare you the necessity of being present, open, and attuned in each moment.

That said, it is easier to be present, open, and attuned when we have some basic level of confidence that we know what we're doing. In spiritually integrated psychotherapy, as in most things, there is no way to prepare ahead for every possible contingency. But there is a framework that is helpful to know, and this framework can be taught.

That is my chief intention in this book: to teach you a framework. Not to tell you everything you'll ever need to know about engaging spirituality in psychotherapy, nor to minimize how important it is to allow your own gifts, sensitivities, and perspectives to affect the way you practice. But to give you the basics, the skeleton, the scaffolding, so that you can do it your own way—the way only you could do it—with confidence that you're working in a trustworthy manner.

WHERE THIS BOOK CAME FROM

This book began in the woods.

I live in the mountains of North Carolina, just outside Asheville, and I spend as much time as possible outside. It's one of my lifelines, to be in the presence of "wild things."[2] I love the deer, the bears, the foxes, and the snakes. I love the peaks, the creeks, and the quiet. I love the birds, their joy, their vulnerability, and the way they fuss when they're annoyed. I love the trees, which are like elders to me. Trees live lives of dignity and service; they've seen it all and survived it; and when it's their time to go, they lie down and begin nourishing the next generation.

I was among the trees, running a favorite trail. It was fall, a sunny afternoon in gold and red late October. It was also a season of grief, four months after a major loss,[3] and as is the way of grief, my outer and inner worlds were being roughly and tenderly rearranged.

I came to a gate that separates the woods from a pasture. I opened it, passed through from the huddle of trees to the open blue sky, and there it was.

Write a book about psychotherapy and spirituality. Write in the same plain, down-to-earth language you use when you talk with clients and friends. Make it practical, not theoretical—you're a therapist, not an academic—and pack it with as much clinical dialogue as you can, so people can hear what this work sounds like and feel less intimidated to try it themselves. Make it adaptable for use with almost any psychotherapy model. And write from your heart. Let it be a book that *feels* spiritual, so the tone of the book might be a match for the topic.

I write an occasional blog, and I've published a few short pieces in religious and literary journals. But I've never felt the tug to write anything "professional." This is partly because the other things I do professionally are plenty satisfying, but mainly because there are already *so many* wonderful books about psychotherapy and spirituality. Here's my personal starting five:

- *Spiritually Integrated Psychotherapy*, by Ken Pargament
- *Encountering the Sacred in Psychotherapy*, by James Griffith and Melissa Elliott Griffith
- *Spiritual and Religious Competencies in Clinical Practice*, by Cassandra Vieten and Shelley Scammell
- *Grace Unfolding*, by Greg Johanson and Ron Kurtz

- *Understanding Pastoral Counseling*, edited by Elizabeth Maynard and Jill Snodgrass

And it's a deep roster. There are many, many other terrific books on this topic.

But none of them is the book I was being prompted to write, a book that says,

- Here's what spiritual conversation actually sounds like in psychotherapy.
- Here are spiritual themes and spiritual issues you'll commonly encounter.
- Here's the essential clinical architecture.
- Here's the sequence and flow of how it happens.
- And oh, by the way, since your own spirituality is part of the therapy process too—the same way your gender, race, social location, and personality style are—here's how to draw upon that aspect of yourself in ethical and skillful ways.

That book, I decided, was worth writing. And here it is.

HOW THIS BOOK IS ORGANIZED

This book is organized into three parts:

1. **An introductory section.** This section includes the present chapter, a couple of chapters about what I mean by "spirituality," and a chapter about the word "God." Think of this first part as an orientation and warm-up for the rest of the book.
2. **A section focused on working with your clients' spirituality.** This section covers what spiritual conversations sound like and how they start, how to assess your

clients spiritually, how to make spiritually oriented interventions, and how to work with spiritual struggles and unhealthy spirituality. Think of this as the nuts-and-bolts how-to section that includes lots of illustrations from my clinical practice. You'll read what I said, when I said it, and why. You'll have to adapt what you say and when you say it to fit your own therapeutic style, but you'll at least have something concrete and specific to work from.

3. **A section focused on you, your spirituality, how you stay aware of it, and how you make use of it.** Lots of therapists tell me they detach themselves as much as they can from their own spirituality, so that they don't inadvertently force their spirituality on their clients. It's impossible to do this completely, of course, but even trying to do this robs these therapists of a rich source of understanding and power. In part 3 I talk about drawing upon your own spiritual history and spiritual beliefs in ethically responsible ways, including working with your spiritual countertransference.

A WORD TO THE WARY

I believe something spiritual is happening every moment in psychotherapy. It's not always explicit, as when a client speaks a clear-cut spiritual word like "God" or "prayer." But if there is a spiritual dimension to human experience—and I believe there is—then it is always present, always affecting our clients' mental health and overall well-being (for better or worse), and always a resource that can be drawn upon to help people stabilize, heal, and change.

If you're reading this book, there's a chance you believe this too. That the spiritual doesn't segregate itself from the rest of human experience in some roped-off spirituality section. That it is integrated and interwoven with all the other dimensions of human experience: mind, body, relationships, and more. And that there are ways of giving attention to the spiritual and working with it that can help people survive the absolute worst life throws at them and change their most intractable habits of thought, feeling, and behavior.

Or maybe you *don't* believe this. Maybe spirituality never made *any* sense to you. Maybe it makes you uncomfortable because it's not part of your background. Or maybe it makes you uncomfortable because it *is* part of your background, and you're still trying to get over it. You'd still like to know what to do when clients introduce spiritual material into their work with you, but you're approaching this book with a bit of wariness.

You might even be wary of the term "spirituality" itself, because in the religious world you're from, "spirituality" is the vague, anything-goes approach of people who aren't really serious about faith, who want to choose the parts they like and ignore the parts they don't. You might be wondering if this book is going to be spiritual enough for you.

However you've come to this book—all aboard and enthusiastic, or uneasy and looking for the first good exit—I'm glad you're here. And if you're among the wary, I'm especially glad. I deeply respect that you're willing to stretch yourself in service of your clients, and I have tried to write this book with respect for you in mind.

By "respect," I do not mean that I have tried to protect you from your uneasiness. I mean more the opposite, that I've tried to give you opportunity here, in this book, to be in the presence of your uneasiness—not to torture you, but to give you strategies for remaining in a conversation that helps another person, even when there's something about that conversation that makes you uneasy, and opportunities to practice those strategies for yourself as you make your way through this book.

Ready? Here we go.

2

....

God

A Word about a Word

IT'S IMPOSSIBLE TO WRITE A BOOK ABOUT PSYCHOTHERAPY AND spirituality without using the word "God." And if it *were* possible to do so, it would be foolish, given how central that word is in so many people's spiritual experience. (The last major survey of religious belief in the United States at the publication time of this book, for example, the Pew Research Center's Religious Landscape Study of 2014, showed that 89 percent of U.S. adults believe in "God or a universal spirit," 63 percent believe in God with "absolute certainty," and 71 percent are Christian.[1])

But the word "God" is a complicated word. It means different things to different people, and it sparks a wide range of associations. So before we go any further, let's talk about God.

THE WORD "GOD" IS A POETIC WORD

There's this beautiful phrase in Buddhism: "the finger pointing at the moon." It comes from a passage in which the Buddha instructs his students to spend more time meditating, observing their actual minds, than listening to his teachings. Your mind, he tells them, is like the luminous moon. My teachings are just a finger pointing to the moon.

All the many names for God are like this. Yahweh, Allah, the Tao, Jesus, Spirit, Brahman, Baha, Higher Power, the Life Force, the Beloved, and more: they are fingers pointing at the moon.

They all convey something true about the Spiritual Ground of Reality, and none of them expresses the Full Truth. They are inspired, soulful stabs at Whatever It Is That'll make a carpenter spend forty days in the wilderness without food; or a prince sit down beneath a bodhi tree and not move until enlightenment strikes; or a criminal who's fled the country return to the scene of his crime, request an audience with the king, and say, "Let my people go"; or a black seamstress not give up her seat on a bus to a white man; or a man step gently but unhesitatingly into the path of a tank in Tiananmen Square; or the adult survivor of childhood abuse ask, "Tell me, what is it you plan to do with your one wild and precious life?"[2] Whatever That is, the That that throws and sows and grows all this grace and grit, That's what we're pointing to when we say the word "God."

Or take all the best words you know: nouns like *love, truth, beauty,* and *grace*; verbs like *touch, breathe, laugh, cry,* and *sing*; adjectives like *tender, fierce, extravagant, hilarious,* and *holy.* That's also what we're pointing to when we say "God."

There are people in all religions, of course, who believe that their particular word for God or understanding of God is "right," or "more right," than others'. And who's to say? But as therapists, our job is not to parse out who's right about God and who's not. Our job is to hear what our clients' experiences with God and beliefs about God mean to them, how they are a resource in their lives, or how our clients might be struggling with this God in some way.

So try this. Try listening to your clients' words about God as poetry, not science, and let those words lead you into deeper connection with the poet in your office.

ATTACHMENT TO GOD, RESISTANCE TO GOD

Some of you reading this may feel quite at home with the word "God." Others of you believe in some sort of Divine Reality, but you are not of the Judeo-Christian-Islamic tradition, and the word "God" is not your word. Or you are of that tradition, but you find the word "God" worn out from overuse or tainted by misuse, and you prefer a different term. Still others of you do not resonate at all with the notion of a theistic universe, and there aren't any words for God that make sense to you.

We can't prove or disprove God, of course, not the way we can prove that "Topeka is in Kansas" or disprove that "the earth is flat." But the God we believe in but can't prove, or don't believe in but can't disprove, always comes with a backstory. Ana-Maria Rizzuto's *Birth of the Living God*, for instance, shows how early-life attachment relationships become blueprints for our adult understandings of God. And later-in-life experiences, too, where God is connected to some cause of kindness or of meanness, also color our relationship with God. Whatever you feel and think about God, there are plenty of good reasons for it. And the same holds for your clients.

That's why, as therapists, it's important not to be overly attached or overly reactive to any particular language about spiritual experience. We want to let our clients teach us their spiritual language, their words for God (or not-God), and we want to respond with the same respect, curiosity, and open heart with which we engage everything else our clients tell us.

This is easy enough when our clients say God (or don't) in a way that resonates with us, but it can be difficult when the God they describe is alien, frightening, or offensive to us. When our reaction to the word "God"—or to the particular way clients use it or don't use it—is so strong that we can't hear it or say it back to them without clenching, fuming, or dissociating, we should consider it a countertransference trailhead to explore with someone we trust. (There is an entire chapter on spiritual countertransference later in the book. Feel free to skip ahead and read it now if you need to.)

For now, though, remember this: when it comes to God, the attitude that will never lead us astray is humility. It is natural, of course, to trust our own experience of God over the experience of others. But we are wise to balance this natural tendency with friendly reminders that our understanding is not the only word and might not be the last word. Whatever your client says about Ultimate Reality, it's a confessional, poetic attempt to say something true about their experience. Try not to be overly attached to the poetry you prefer or overly reactive to the poetry you don't.

NEVERTHELESS, I'M STILL GONNA SAY "GOD"

"God" is not God's actual name, but I am still going to use the word "God" freely in this book. I will sometimes use terms that are religiously and philosophically more neutral, like "the sacred" or "the transcendent." These are the words more customarily used in books about psychotherapy and spirituality, and I will occasionally use them too. I'll also use some of the more popular inclusive phrases like "Higher Power" and "Life Force," or poetic words like "Love" and "the Universe."

But most often, in reference to the sacred, I will just use the word "God." I'm doing this for several reasons:

- My intention in this book, as much as I can, is to write the way your clients actually talk. And "God" is the word most people use and resonate with, positively or negatively. I'll bet even your most secular clients do not say, "O My Transcendence!" when they're surprised, or "O Highest of All Human Values!" when they have an orgasm.

- The word "God" connotes the sense of personhood that many of your clients experience in their spiritual lives. Words like "sacred" and "transcendent," while less particular and less likely to rub anyone the wrong way, are a bit dry and academic. They sound like ideas more than people. God is not a person, of course, not in the way that you and I are persons, but for many people, God is "like" a person, sort of, and I'm wanting to write in the personal way your clients really talk.

- I trust you, the reader, to understand the word "God" poetically and to translate it into whatever images have integrity for you and your clients.

- Finally, if you do have a countertransference reaction to the word "God," I'm wanting you to have it now, while you're reading this book and can talk about it with someone, not later, while you're with clients who are telling you about what matters most to them.

On we go, then. With God.

3

Spirituality, Spiritually

WHAT IS SPIRITUALITY, ANYWAY?

That's a fair question, especially for a book about psychotherapy and spirituality. And I'm going to answer it two ways.

In the next chapter I'll talk about spirituality in a theoretical way. I'll give you a definition, describe the relationship between spirituality and other dimensions of human experience, talk about the conspicuous and inconspicuous ways spirituality appears, and more.

But first, in this chapter, I want to begin the way spirituality begins: not as a concept but as an experience. Before it ever becomes as an abstract *-ality* that gets defined in a book, spirituality is something that happens. It's something we experience, something that affects us, something we feel. And I want to start there, bringing you as close as I can to the breath and bone and marrow of spirituality.

To do this, to give you a feel for the breadth and depth and spirit of spirituality, I wrote up a list of questions and looked for opportunities to ask them of friends, family, colleagues, and clients:

- What does spirituality feel like?
- What do you notice when a spiritual experience is happening?
- What is it about an experience that makes you call it "spiritual"?
- If you had to describe spirituality to someone who had no idea what it is, what would you say?
- When and where do spiritual experiences happen for you?
- How do they affect you?

These questions sparked some amazing conversations—I honestly can't recommend this exercise highly enough—and the result, as you might imagine, was a beautiful, illuminating, sprawling, holy mess. In the rest of this chapter, I'll reach into that holy mess and pull out descriptions of spiritual experiences. I'll present them like a collage you might have made in art class, rather than the periodic table of elements you learned in chemistry, not because I'm too lazy to organize them, but because a collage is more in keeping with the undomesticated, unpredictable nature of spiritual experience. Some of what's in the collage are the exact words of others. Some are composites. Some are my own.

My small hope is that what follows conveys some of the feel of spirituality. My larger hope is that it stirs you to reflect on your own experience of spirituality.

DESCRIPTIONS OF SPIRITUALITY

"You know that feeling when you're in the woods and you hear birds singing, and you stop to listen? The way not just your ears but your whole body gets still and expectant? You know there's a song out there, and you're waiting for it to return, and you can't see the singer, and you don't control the singer. And inwardly you're partly asking for it and partly just waiting for it without asking? That's what a spiritual experience feels like to me. That quiet, expectant stillness. That getting my own busyness and clumsiness out of the way, and listening for the song in the woods."

"Sometimes I'm in the flow of things. The wind is at my back. Everything's clicking. And it feels like God is saying, 'Yes.' And sometimes the wind is in my face, and it's a strong wind. And everything's an effort. 'Here, pull this plow through this field. And while you're at it, also carry this bag of bricks.' And God's saying, 'Keep going. This is hard but it's right.' And sometimes it's like running into a wall. *Bam!* Door closed. Game over. Turn around. Not this. Something else. And God's saying, 'No. Not this. Not now.' And the feeling I have is . . . what's a decent word for it? . . . Clarity. Deep knowing. Like I'm getting to know something extremely important, and it's hard to know it, but I'm getting help to know it."

"Spiritual experience, for me, is being in the presence of something unseen. Like right now, right this second, there's all this air around me. I don't see it, but it's there. It's touching my skin. I'm breathing it in. If I get up and walk, I'll be walking through it. Whatever I do, it's there. I live my life in it. It's in me. I'm in it. Spiritual experience is like feeling that unseen air."

"One of the ways I've been affected by spiritual experiences is that I believe everything and everyone are connected. I don't just mean that we're connected like links in a chain. I mean we're all made of the same thing. Materially speaking, everything is made of whatever it was that exploded in the big bang. Spiritually speaking, everything is coming from the continuous consciousness of God. Sometimes I'll look at a tree, or mist on a field, or a complete stranger, or my husband, or even someone from history long ago, and I have this deep sense that we're just different arrangements of the same material and energy."

"I'm part of a small group Bible study through my church. We meet every week. We eat a simple meal together. We read the Bible and talk about how it's speaking to us this week. People say things they're learning, things they're grateful for, things they're struggling with. Then we pray. And some weeks, not every week, but some weeks when we pray, it feels like a cloud has come down and settled upon us. My breath changes. It feels like the cloud is breathing for me, like I'm on a respirator or something. Like we're all on this respirator together, being breathed into together, connected with each other in this cloud. I guess that's what they call the Holy Spirit."

"What's spiritual to me are those times when I get a sense of 'Wow!' For a long time, it was music—a group of people playing totally separate notes that could combine to generate a wave of sonic 'feeling' that could transport me. After I moved to Asheville, I have found it most often in nature—a mountain vista, a bubbling stream, moss-covered rocks, gnarled trees, delicate flowers. Nowadays, that's usually where I get that internal sigh, 'Ahhhh,' or that 'Wow!'"

"I have this statue of Buddha on a bookshelf at home. I pass by it several times a day, and sometimes

I don't even notice it. But sometimes I pause, and I look at him, and he looks at me, and I feel connected with his stillness, and his acceptance, and his wisdom, and his laughter. And we smile at each other, and my heart feels warm. I grew up Methodist, and there's this thing John Wesley[1] said about being with Jesus and feeling his heart strangely warmed. I still feel sort of connected to Jesus, but I think he's handed me off for Buddha to take care of."

"Sometimes when I'm feeling spiritual, I feel very small. Like, there's how many stars in the galaxy? Two hundred billion? And our galaxy is one of how many other galaxies? Another 100 billion? So the earth is the tiniest, tiniest speck in this unfathomably massive universe. And you and I, we're just these tiny, tiny specks on a tiny, tiny speck. And I like feeling small like this. It doesn't feel scary. It doesn't feel like I'm unimportant. It just takes the pressure off. You go through life feeling like everything you do is so important. There's so much riding on it. At least, that's how I go through life, a lot of the time. Maybe I should go see a therapist, huh? But spirituality is when I know the truth that I'm just a speck on a speck, and soon I'll be gone, and for me, that's liberating. It's like cooling off after I've been really hot."

"God has these signals he sends me, to let me know he's with me. Certain colors, certain sounds, certain words. I see them or hear them outside myself, or inside myself, just in my own mind. And when I get those signals, sometimes it changes me instantly, and I feel calmer and stronger. And sometimes it takes a bit, but at least I know God is with me, and calmer and stronger are on the way."

"The times that feel most spiritual to me are when I feel at home in my body and at home in my surroundings, at the same time. I'm present in both. I'm present *with* both. There's this sense of connectedness. There's a Heschel quote that I love: 'I *am* what is not mine.'[2] I'm so connected to all this that I don't own or control that I *am* that. And what I'm at home in isn't a permanent home. What's happening might be profoundly beautiful or profoundly horrible. But either way, it's a temporary home. Joy, grief, fear, anger—none of it's binding, none of it's permanent."

"There's an old motel here that's been turned into a shelter for veterans who are homeless. I go there on weekends and help cook breakfast. I don't know that I feel all that spiritual when I'm doing it. I'm mostly just focused on whatever I'm doing: cracking eggs, stirring grits, whatever. But I do think it's spiritual. Jesus said that when you feed somebody who's hungry or visit somebody who's sick, you're feeding him or visiting him. So that's my way of seeing Jesus on the weekend."

"One time I woke up in the middle of the night, and there was music coming out of my heart. I'm not kidding. And I was awake. I wasn't dreaming, I'm certain. But if I was, really, who cares? The music—it was several voices and a banjo, and maybe a guitar, and definitely a glockenspiel. I was lying on my back, and it was pouring up out of my heart. It felt a little like I was part of the singing, but mostly it was like the music was being made somewhere else and being channeled through me. Can you imagine? That was a spiritual experience for me, and that's what spirituality means to me: just being a channel for God, being part of God, being part of the eternal song."

"I think of discouragement and despair as spiritual experiences. I don't know if you're hearing that from anyone else. But they're just as spiritual to me as joy and hope. When I think about how twenty-five thousand people die every day from hunger, or that there are 65 million people on earth right now who are refugees, or that somebody's gonna walk into a school or shopping mall this month and shoot another twenty people, or that the girl who rings up my groceries is going home to a father or a boyfriend who hits her, and there's not a damn thing I can do about it—that just really gets to me. And sometimes I feel mad, but mostly I just feel hopeless and powerless and paralyzed about those things. But somehow that feels spiritual to me too. Just to see all that crap, to witness it, and be affected by it, and not turn away from it. Even if I don't know what to do about any of it. Just to witness it and feel horrible about it. Spirituality isn't all laughter and light, you know."

"Being with my father while he died was the most spiritual moment of my life."

"I find a sense of the spiritual singing in the choir at church—the resonance of my voice in my chest, the tones coming out of my mouth, and the merging of those tones with those of the other singers."

"I regularly attend Al-Anon twelve-step meetings, and through that I practice continually reconnecting to my Higher Power. I think we as humans have a tendency to disconnect from our Higher Power to do all the other things in our lives. Going to Al-Anon helps me remember I'm not alone and it's not all up to me."

"My father was a strong spiritual presence in my life. And in the years since he died, there are times when I feel his presence with me. I feel it physically. There's like a presence and a tingle. I can feel the air change. I remember doing Outward Bound when I was in my forties, and there's a twenty-four-hour solo experience. I was so scared to spend the night alone in the woods. But when it got dark, I felt him come settle in beside me, and I slept through the night without waking."

"I had a spiritual experience the first time I used psychedelic drugs. I experienced a sense of oneness with everything—people, plants, rocks, trees, the clouds—all of creation—that literally 'blew my mind' and all my preconceptions of me as separate. It probably—no, truly—changed my way of thinking and feeling."

"I have a meditation app on my phone. It's partly a timer, but it also tells me how many other people across the world are using this app and meditating right this minute. I don't know if you meditate or not, but sometimes it's a very peaceful experience, and other times it's an absolute loony bin. So especially on the days when my meditation time is crazy-town, it means something to me to know that there are other people doing this thing, and maybe somewhere in this web there's somebody else's calm I might be tapping into."

"Right now my spiritual experience is one of great pain and frustration. I used to feel a pretty strong connection with God, but the past few years I don't. I want to feel him with me so bad. I try to pray, and that lasts for about thirty seconds, because I don't feel any connection at all. I'm reaching for God so hard, and nothing's reaching back."

"Several years ago, I was taking a one-week grad-school elective (on spirituality, coincidentally). One student arrived late to the first class because she had just flown back from a family vacation in Turkey. She gave everyone in the class a rock from Turkey. Now, I knew Turkey existed, and I could have located it on a map, but other than that, I'd never given much thought to the country. But this simple gesture made me curious about the country, and I Googled it during the week. The class wrapped up on a Friday, and the very next weekend, I met a friend of a friend who came to this country thirty-plus years ago from Turkey. I ended up giving him the souvenir rock, which was very meaningful and emotional to him. Long story short, he and I have been married now for three years. To me, that is not coincidence. It was destiny, fate, divine intervention—whatever you want to call it. But that is the spiritual at work."

"Spiritual experience for me is about being connected with my heart. I don't mean just the organ in my chest, though that's part of it. It's also my eyes, ears, guts, arms, legs, genitals, brain—everything. Heart is the place in me where mind, body, and spirit all gather together. It's where I experience emotion, intuition, and deep knowing. There's somebody who talks about prayer being moving from your head to your heart,[3] and I resonate with that so much. It's not always easy for me to make that move. I live in my head a lot. Making lists. Keeping time. Racing around. And sometimes I find my heart is so tight and guarded and hard. But sometimes I can touch my heart with my breath, very lightly, like a petal of a flower falling on water, and sometimes that softens my heart or opens it. Sometimes I can feel love flowing out to the world through my heart. Other times my heart feels like a mirror that can reflect love in different directions and send it out to people in the room with me."

"Every morning I read Scripture—usually it's the Bible, but sometimes I read the Tao Te Ching or something from the Buddha. Then I meditate for twenty minutes, and I always end my meditation with the Twenty-third Psalm. I think that psalm has the whole spiritual life in it. There's wanting and not-wanting, resting, nature, pastures and water, stillness, fearing and not fearing, death, valleys, shadow, evil, comfort, a table of food, enemies, anointing, goodness, mercy, and dwelling. I mean, what else is there?"

"It's hard to pull out 'spiritual' experiences because spiritual feels like the fabric of life to me. Trying to pull out one thread as an example isn't really possible—you lose the whole. It's so woven in. Drinking coffee, washing dishes, writing a letter, stacking wood, driving and listening to the radio—it's all spiritual."

CONCLUSION

The last line of the Gospel of John goes like this: "There are also many other things that Jesus did; if every one of them were written down, I suppose that the world itself could not contain the books that would be written."[4] And that's true of this collage. We could keep adding to it for the rest of our lives, and it would never be finished.

I hope that some of the words above make sense to you and that some don't. Spiritual experience isn't all supposed to make sense.

I also hope they've set off a chain reaction of associations, memories, and visceral rumblings in you—an even more beautiful, illuminating, sprawling, holy mess—and that you're adding your own experience to the collage.

And finally, I hope the spirit of this chapter infects the rest of the book and your experience of it—including the next chapter, where we consider spirituality in a bit more rational and orderly fashion.

4

Spirituality, Conceptually

In CHAPTER 3 WE APPROACHED SPIRITUALITY IN AN IMPRES-
sionistic way. That was a spirituality *collage*. Here we'll consider spirituality in a more conceptual and organized way. This
chapter is spirituality *college*.

There are tens of thousands of academic books and articles
about spirituality. They examine spirituality and neurobiology,
spirituality and psychology, spirituality and sociology, spirituality and health, spirituality and social change, spirituality and
literature, spirituality and art, and on and on. There are thousands more just on the topic of spirituality and psychotherapy.
If you read some of those—and I hope you will—your appreciation for the complexity, diversity, and expanse of spirituality
will only increase.

We can't cover all that, though. What's here are a few points
I think are most salient for the work we do as therapists.

A DEFINITION FOR THERAPISTS

If this were a book for scholars, or for therapists who would
do their work better if they talked more like scholars, I would

reference several of my favorite definitions of spirituality and then write something like this:

> Spirituality refers to the multiple, interrelated, and cul-turally diverse dynamics by which humans experience the sacred or transcendent dimension of life. These multiple, interrelated, and culturally diverse dynam-ics include the desire for transcendent experience, the substance of such experience (beliefs, values, emotions, somatic experience, behaviors, interactive-relational-social elements), and the processes and practices that make possible or facilitate such expe-rience. The sacred or transcendent dimension of life includes theistic-oriented and non-theistic-oriented awareness of realities larger than the individual self, awareness that comes via experiences with the divine, with others, with nature, with art, etc.

But this is a book for therapists, like you. And while you probably understand that definition, and while it might satisfy readers of an academic journal, it's not how clients talk in your office, and it's not how *you* talk in your office.

Here's a definition of spirituality that's a bit more office-ready:

> Spirituality is all the ways you and God relate to each other.

Remember, please, that I'm using the word "God" intention-ally in this book (rather than a designation like "the sacred") not to advance a particular spiritual point of view but to speak the way your clients are most likely to speak. Also, remember that the word "God" here is a poetic word. You can replace it with whatever word you or the particular client in your office might resonate with—Allah, Krishna, Jesus, Buddha Nature, Higher Power, the Life Force, the Universe. Just let it be a word that would warm the space between you and your client, something with some color, texture, and oomph.

THE WAY YOU AND GOD RELATE

I'm saying "spirituality is all the ways you and God relate to each other," rather than "all the ways you relate to God" or "all the ways God relates to you," because I want to highlight the two-way, relational quality of spiritual experience.

Ken Pargament, whom I greatly admire, defines spirituality as "the search for the sacred."[1] But that definition references a one-way relationship—*us searching for God*—and spirituality is also about *God searching for us*. It's like the lines from the poet Gregory Orr:

> As with lovers:
>
> When it's right you can't say
> Who is kissing Whom.[2]

Spirituality is a back-and-forth, active-and-receptive, seek-and-be-sought thing. (Also, sometimes, it's a seek-and-feel-nothing-back thing, or a be-sought-and-avoid thing.[3])

Also, like all relationships, a spiritual relationship can be a healthy one that increases our capacities for love, freedom, creativity, connection, morality, courage, and calmness. Or it can be an unhealthy one, contributing to experiences of anxiety, despair, isolation, self-hatred, other-hatred, and violence. (We'll talk more about healthy and unhealthy spirituality in the chapters on spiritual assessment and spiritual interventions.)

YOU, SPECIFICALLY

Spirituality is a relationship, and every relationship is different.

You've probably heard the phrase "Like all others, like some others, like no others."[4] It describes how we humans are simultaneously both alike and different from one another. It's true about us in every way I can think of, including spiritually.

When I introduce this idea in a workshop, I ask participants to look around the room and notice how different we all are physically. We're all people, so there are similarities. Nobody gets mistaken for a motorcycle or a giraffe. But we're all different too—different colors, different body shapes, different eyes, noses, mouths, arms, and legs.

Then I ask, "If it's true that we're all a bit different physically, isn't it likely that we're all a bit different spiritually too?"

"The way you and God relate to each other" is unique for every "you." You got a feel for that in the last chapter, and it's important to remember: everyone has a unique spiritual fingerprint, we don't all fit into the same spiritual box, and God connects with each of us in unique ways.

Also remember that *not feeling connected to God* is a way of being in relationship with God—you heard that in the last chapter too—and there needs to be room in our understanding of spirituality for spiritual dryness, emptiness, forsakenness, meaninglessness, disbelief, and disinterest.

This respect for spiritual diversity is an absolute essential for working with spirituality in psychotherapy. It's not just that our codes of ethics say we should not promote a particular spiritual perspective. More importantly, we will get further with our clients if we understand all of them as unique spiritual people, with whom God has unique ways of connecting, and whose lives can be better when they recognize their spiritual uniqueness and use it as a resource.

We therapists have our own spiritual beliefs and practices too, and we can use them to inform our work with clients and for self-care. (That's what part 3 of this book is about.) But if we want to maximize our clinical effectiveness and do right by our clients, we will try to understand *their* unique relationship with God.

SPIRITUALITY AND RELIGION

Spirituality is closely related to religion, and we encounter both in psychotherapy. Everyday people sometimes use these words interchangeably and sometimes in contrast (as in, "I'm spiritual but not religious"). The psychotherapy and spirituality literature recognizes the overlap between spirituality and religion but generally distinguishes them in this way:

- *Spirituality* refers more to an inward, personal experience.
- *Religion* refers more to a social, institutional experience.

To say a bit more, spirituality is about meaning and connection, the innate human impulse to make sense of our lives and to connect with something "beyond sense" (the transcendent). Religion is about meaning and connection in a group, like the Roman Catholic Church or the Zen Center down the street.

Spirituality is the subjective experience of an individual. Religion is the shared beliefs, values, and practices of a community. Here is a representative quote, from James Griffith: "Spirituality has more to do with the interior psychological lives of individuals, while religion is more manifest in group life and society as a whole."[5]

That's the view from ten thousand feet. Closer to the ground, of course, there's a lot of nuance. We can't really separate the inward and psychological from the social and cultural. Our experiences in groups and cultures shape our personal experiences, and our personal experiences shape groups and cultures. In reality, the line between spirituality and religion is a fuzzy one, and the question of which is the larger construct—does spirituality come first and give rise to religion, or does religion come first and give rise to spirituality?—a question academics sometimes argue about, cannot ultimately be answered.

Neither can we say for sure which is "better." Some people observe the abuses of organized religion, or the way we can participate in group activities without being personally, experientially engaged, and assert that spirituality is "better" than religion. Others note the way personal spirituality can be self-serving, shallow, isolated, and lacking in accountability, and say that religion is "better" than spirituality. But these arguments tend to stand on best-case and worst-case examples that support the bias of whoever's speaking, and most of the literature recognizes the ambiguous strengths and weakness of both spirituality and religion.

These overlaps and nuances noted, let me say a bit more about the big-picture differences between the two.

Religion is a "like some others" thing. In religion, there are common customs, a common language, a particular way of dressing, a special place to gather, and special rituals performed, all of which reinforce the beliefs, values, and practices of the group. There's a tribal quality to organized religion that gives us a sense of identity and belonging.

Spirituality is a "like no other" thing. It has an interior, experiential, organic, in-the-moment quality that is unique to the person experiencing it. It is difficult, if not impossible, to organize, and it doesn't always look "religious."

Here's an example: a man praying the Al Chet (confession of sins) at Yom Kippur services, aloud and with other worshippers, is participating in a religious experience. That same man, praying the Al Chet, taking the words to heart, and being inwardly moved by them, is having a religious and a spiritual experience. A different man, attending the service because his mother wants him to, saying the words of the Al Chet while actually thinking about how to fix the leaky faucet when he gets home, is having a religious experience but not a spiritual one. And a woman walking by the synagogue, smelling freshly fallen pine needles, feeling the wind, noticing a palpable-but-deeper-than-words connection with the trees and the wind, and feeling her heart warmed and eased at this moment, is having a spiritual experience but not a religious one.

Here's another example, from a clinical context. A client who goes to her garden to connect with God when she's stressed is drawing upon a personal spiritual resource. A client who calls her minister in a time of crisis is using a community-based religious resource.

To summarize what I've said so far and make clear how I'm using the terms in this book:

- *Spirituality* is all the ways you and God relate to each other—all the ways: inward and outward, visible and invisible, solitary and shared.
- *Religion* is when the way you and God relate is connected to a community of shared beliefs, values, and practices.
- *Spirituality happens sometimes in connection to religion, and sometimes apart from religion.*

BODY WORDS

Etymologically, "spirituality" and "religion" are both body words, and this is clinically rather significant.

The word "spirit" comes from the Latin *spiritus*, which means breath. It's the same root that gives us words like "respiration" and "inspiration." In the biblical languages, Hebrew and Greek, the word that means spirit also means breath and wind.[6] Spirituality, then, is a relationship that animates us (like breath does) and moves us (like wind). It's about being breathed by the Breath and blown by the Wind. It's an inhale-exhale, active-receptive, move-and-be-moved relationship.

Like any relationship, spirituality can be good for you or bad for you. If the *spiritus* you're breathing is rich in oxygen and clean of pollution—if the God you're in relationship with is loving and kind—your spirituality will be healthy. It will make you a better person. It will bring you energy and power, or calmness and peace, as you need it, and it will move you to relate to others with love and kindness. And vice versa. If the *spiritus* you're breathing is toxic—if your God is harsh and hateful—your spirituality will be unhealthy. It will hurt you and hurt others.

The word "religion" is also a body word. It comes from the Latin *religare* and the root word *lig*, as in "ligament." This gives a good feel for the deep meaning of religion: it reconnects things.

I like the way the Franciscan priest Richard Rohr talks about this point. He says that religion helps reconnect four major splits that people make again and again, to varying degrees:

1. We split from our shadow self and pretend to be our idealized self.
2. We split our mind from our body and soul and pretend to live in our mind.
3. We split life from death and try to live our life without any "death."
4. We split ourselves from other selves and try to live apart, superior, and separate.[7]

Unhealthy religion tends to reinforce these splits, but healthy religion re-*ligs* them. It reconnects these fragments and brings about a transformation in human consciousness and behavior.

The word "yoga" also expresses this reconnecting, uniting quality of healthy religion. Yoga means "union" or "integration." (It has a similar meaning to the soundalike word "yoke.") In Hindu practice, the goal of yoga is to bring us back into union with God and with all aspects of ourselves.[8]

BIO-PSYCHO-SOCIAL-SPIRITUAL

The body-rootedness of the words "spirituality" and "religion" reminds us that spirit is inseparable from body. But spirit is also inseparable from "psyche" and from the relational and social fabric of our lives.

A phrase you'll hear a lot in the world of psychotherapy and spirituality is "bio-psycho-social-spiritual." This mashup phrase points to the way people comprise these four dimensions: bodies, minds, webs of relationships and social forces, and spirit. Considering all four dimensions helps us understand the complexity of human health and illness, and it's important to assess our clients' strengths and struggles in all four areas.

But these four areas are separable from one another only in theory. In an actual human life, mental, physical, social, and spiritual are all happening at the same time. If one of your clients says, "I felt the presence of God," and you ask him to tell you more about it, he might say, "I felt a calmness in my chest" (describing his body), "I felt a sense of peace, and I wasn't angry anymore" (describing his psychological state), and "I stopped yelling at my brother" (describing a social-relational dynamic).

So even though this book focuses on the dimension of "spirituality," let's be clear that what we're talking about is a part of life that can't really be separated out from the rest of it. A spiritual experience is also a physical experience, a psychological experience, and a social experience.

IS EVERYONE SPIRITUAL?

In a word: yes. I believe everyone is spiritual. Every*thing* is spiritual. The whole world, people included, is a resonating incarnation of the Being that exploded into being 13.8 billion years ago. Spirit is part of everything, and everything is part of Spirit. Or as it's said in Hinduism, "Tat Tvam Asi" (Thou art that).

I can't prove this, of course, but it definitely informs the way I live in the world and the way I practice psychotherapy. I believe that every one of my clients is made in God's image, everyone is an expression of God's spirit, everyone always knows which way the Light is, everyone has inward access to all God's qualities—compassion, wisdom, courage, and the like. None of these qualities needs to be imported or installed by me as the therapist. They are already there. I must simply learn to see them and conspire with them. ("Conspire" is another of those breath-spirit words. It means literally "to breathe with.")

I do not argue with people who say they aren't spiritual, and I feel no need to convince anyone to think of themselves that way. What would be the point of that? But I do believe that, conscious of it or not, everyone is spiritual. People don't have to be conscious of oxygen to breathe, or believe in the unconscious to dream. It's like the story of two fish swimming. One says, "Man! The water is so wet today!" The other says, "What's water?"[9]

We're all free to regard or disregard the spiritual dimension of our lives. We're free to identify as spiritual or not. But, in my view, we have no choice about whether we *are* spiritual beings, any more than we do about whether we are physical, psychological, or social beings.

You can work with spirituality in psychotherapy even if you disagree with me on this point. I know lots of therapists who work with spirituality in psychotherapy because spirituality is a construct within which their client lives, but who do not live in such a construct themselves. If this is you—if you are a therapist interested in your clients' spirituality but who does not have a spiritual sensibility yourself—there are tools in the rest of the book that will serve you. But some of what follows, perhaps much of what follows, does reflect my belief that everyone is, at heart, a spiritual being, and that our spiritual understanding of people can usefully inform the ways we offer help.

EXPLICIT AND IMPLICIT SPIRITUALITY

Everything might *be* spiritual—as I believe—but everything is not *explicitly* spiritual. Some things are recognizable as spiritual only by those who see them that way.

Explicit spirituality refers to things that are obviously spiritual. They might be obvious to an outside observer: someone saying the word "God" aloud, people sitting in group meditation, or someone wearing a cross on a necklace. Or those things might be obvious only to the person having the experience: someone praying or meditating, drawing on faith to make a moral choice, or asking help from deceased ancestors. An outside observer wouldn't necessarily know anything spiritual is going on, but the person having the experience thinks of it in an explicitly spiritual way, and if she told you about it in your office, she would identify it that way.

Implicit spirituality refers to experiences of spiritual significance that don't show up wearing a "spirituality" name tag. It's when the spiritual quality of an experience is embedded but not explicit. Watching a sunset or sharing a smile with a stranger are examples of implicit spiritual experiences. So are moments of gratitude and forgiveness, or experiences of compassion, humility, and agency. As therapists with a spiritual orientation, we might hear spiritual dynamics implicit in the experiences our clients are describing (or experiences they are having right now, in the office with us), even if our clients are not thinking of them in that way. We would not force this understanding on our clients; we might not even mention it, but it might inform our work with them all the same. (I will say more about this in later chapters.)

Many implicit spiritual experiences occur at the fuzzy intersection of the psychological and the spiritual. We often call them psychospiritual, and they include experiences like the sampling below:

Acceptance	Emptiness	Liberation
Aloneness	Envy	Longing
Anger	Forgiveness	Love
Anxiety	Generosity	Lust
Awe	Gratitude	Oppression
Bitterness	Greed	Pain
Burden	Guilt	Patience
Comfort	Hatred	Pride
Connection	Hope	Purpose
Contentment	Joy	Shame
Creativity	Kindness	Trust
Despair	Laziness	Wonder

Notice that some of these represent experiences not everyone considers spiritual. For some, the experience of greed is purely and simply psychological. But for many others, it's a mix of psychological and spiritual. Notice also that some of these words point to experiences we'd consider positive, while others are experiences of anguish or struggle. Spirituality includes the full spectrum of human experience.

For our purposes, as therapists attuned to the spiritual dimension of our clients' lives, it's important that we recognize the broad range of human experiences that can have spiritual resonance. When a client says something like, "I feel so grateful" or "I feel trapped" or "My life is a desert right now," we need eyes to see and ears to hear the implicit spiritual meaning in those statements. We can have an important spiritual conversation with a client without either of us saying a single explicitly spiritual word.

SPIRITUAL EXPERIENCES AND SPIRITUAL MEANING

I've now staked a rather large territory for spirituality. The spiritual realm, I've said, includes everything and everyone. Sometimes it's explicit. Sometimes it's implicit. But everything is spiritual.

Even so, some experiences just *feel* more spiritual than others. There's an energy to them, a flavor, a certain quality, and we got a sense of that in the last chapter.

Spiritual experiences are often connected with experiences like wonder, gratitude, humility, generosity, stillness, connectedness, resonance, peace, comfort, and love. They can occur in explicitly religious settings, like a Bible study, and in settings not explicitly religious, like a veterans' shelter. They often happen in nature and with music. They sometimes involve delightful synchronicities, and other times horrific ordeals. People having spiritual experiences often feel they are being supported or guided by unseen spiritual beings: God, angels, loved ones who have died, and other spirit-guides.

Spiritual experiences help people wake up to the fullness and truth of their own lives and of the world around. The word "Buddha" means literally, "I am awake." God called Samuel to wake up.[10] Jesus tells his disciples to "stay awake."[11]

Spirituality is also about the search for meaning, the hunger to understand life and how to live it well. It's about living into answers to big questions like these:

- Who am I?
- Where did I come from?

- What am I here for?
- How do I deal with impermanence and other forms of change?
- How do I deal with suffering?
- What does it mean that we die? And what happens after we die?
- Are we the highest power in the universe? Or is there a Higher Power?
- If there is a Higher Power, is It benevolent? Does It care about us?
- What do I do about the mistakes I make? How do I atone for the hurts I cause?
- What makes for a good day?
- What makes for a good life?
- What makes life worth living?[12]
- What do I really want?

Questions like these don't have single answers or answers carved in stone. They have multiple answers, most of them in clay. But they are the questions that give our lives a pulse and a direction, and they are the questions people bring with them to psychotherapy.

CONCLUSION

In these first four chapters, I have offered a condensed introduction to spirituality and why it is important in the work of psychotherapy. As I have described it, spirituality is an elemental and continuous part of the human condition, as elemental and continuous as physical, psychological, and social experiences. Also, like these domains, spirituality takes different shape in different people and expresses itself in diverse, even paradoxical, ways: belief and unbelief, ecstasy and despair, living and dying, and the like. Sometimes human spirituality is explicit and obvious. Other times it is implicit and visible only to those with eyes to see. But there is no human experience that is not also a spiritual experience, and there is no conversation in psychotherapy that is not also a spiritual conversation.

There are entire libraries devoted to these topics, and what I've written in these few pages is but a scratch of the surface. I encourage you to dive more deeply, beneath the surface, with support beyond this book. But in the interest of giving you something clinically practical and manageably readable, I am now leaving this introductory space, with many things yet unsaid, and moving on to the psychotherapy room itself.

PART TWO

Working with
Your Client's Spirituality

5

How Spiritual Conversation Begins

WELCOME TO PART 2. THE FIVE CHAPTERS IN THIS PART OF THE book are the meat-and-potatoes—or, if you prefer, the tempeh-and-quinoa—chapters. Here you'll learn specific how-tos for working with your clients' spirituality.

In successive chapters, we'll talk about spiritual assessment, working with healthy spiritual resources, spiritual struggles, and harmful spirituality. But before any of that can happen, a spiritual conversation must begin. This chapter describes how spiritual conversations get started and what you, as the therapist, can do to recognize, invite, and nourish them without imposing your own spiritual beliefs and values.

You might be wondering: Why a whole chapter about how spiritual conversations begin? Don't they begin like all other conversations? Someone says something. Someone else says something back. What's the big deal?

I offer you two answers. First, the way we start sets the tone and makes the way for all that follows. To quote the great Mary Poppins, "Well begun is half done."

Second, we want to begin spiritual conversations in a way that does not impose our spiritual beliefs and values on our clients. Imposition can happen in egregiously unethical ways—a client discloses an affair, and the therapist says, "You know that's a sin, don't you?" But it can also happen in subtle ways that tilt the therapeutic frame and limit what's possible in the therapeutic encounter. Even the relatively neutral word "spirituality" is not entirely neutral. For some clients, spirituality is the watered down, wishy-washy inferior of full-blooded, orthodox religion. So we can ask a fairly innocent question—"Is spirituality important to you?"—and potentially have imposed an assumption and caused a therapeutic rupture.

We want to open a wide and welcoming space where transformational experiences can happen for our clients, and we don't want our own understandings to constrict that space. So if there are ways to begin spiritual conversation that keep our own spiritual assumptions from getting in the way of something amazing happening, we want to do that. Right?

Thus, this chapter on how to begin.

SAFETY FIRST

Stephen Porges, developer of Polyvagal Theory, says that the most important quality of a therapist is the capacity to help other people feel safe.[1] This is true for all aspects of therapy, but it's especially true when people are talking about things that are sacred to them. When it comes to spiritual matters, people can be passionate, defensive, rigid, and sometimes even aggressive. They can also be tentative, reserved, embarrassed, and reluctant to say much of anything. If we want to encourage spiritual conversation in therapy, we need to be good at helping people feel they can be themselves with us, speak what's true for them, and know they won't be met with judgment or some other form of aggression.

We do lots of things to send these safety signals. I'll mention two. First, we use our bodies, particularly our faces and voices, to let others know we mean them good and not harm. People take their safety cues from nonverbal signals way more than from actual words. When our own bodies are grounded and at ease; when our faces are warm, open, and receptive; when our voices are fluid and smooth, people intuit that we are not a threat to them, and they feel safe to engage us without the full arsenal of their defenses.

It doesn't always work, of course. No matter how good we are at signaling safety, there will always be people who aren't able to trust us. People carry trauma wounds and attachment wounds that require a variety of defensive strategies, including being guarded and slow to trust. For some clients, getting to the place of feeling appropriately safe is the *entire goal* of therapy, not the starting point. But we should do what we can with our words and our bodies—especially our bodies—to help people feel safe.

A second way to help people feel safe around us is by cultivating certain spiritual qualities that we carry inside us. These are "person of the therapist" attributes that people intuitively sense in us. They include qualities like these:

Love. Also known as *compassion, care,* and *kindness,* love conveys tenderness, warmth, and "I want good for you."

Humility. Personally, professionally, and spiritually, humility knows that we don't have all the answers, that we don't usually know what's best, and that we get further therapeutically from a posture of not-knowing than from one of all-knowing.

Humanness. We're persons first, therapists second. We all bleed. We all feel longing, joy, fear, sorrow, lust, weariness, contentment, anger, and more. Particularly when you and your client have spiritual differences, your authenticity and humanness are what will connect you and help create safety for your client.

Curiosity. There is more power in asking than there is in assuming. I think the opposite of curiosity is prejudice.

Courage. Real courage is not the puffed-up, steel-jawed machismo that tries to hide fear. Real courage is the willingness to show up as a real person, to offer ourselves in love to another person, to be in relation across difference, to get to the edge of our comfort zone and stretch a little further.

Humor. Therapy is serious business, but there's also a playfulness to the experimenting, improvising, and fumbling around that we do. There are miles of heartache on the road to healing, for sure, but put your ear to the door of most therapy offices and you'll hear plenty of laughing too. Life is funny, people are funny, and when people get together and get real, somehow, merry gets made.

I believe these are qualities we all have, they are always in us, and our role is not to create them but to soften whatever barriers might keep them from flowing freely in us. But however they get there, I hope you sense these qualities—and more—inside yourself. I also hope you know in your bones how important they are for meaningful spiritual conversations to happen in therapy.

HOW SPIRITUAL CONVERSATIONS BEGIN

Safety established, spiritual conversations in psychotherapy begin in one of these ways:

1. The client says something explicitly spiritual, and the therapist responds.
2. The client says something implicitly spiritual, and the therapist responds.

3. The therapist asks in a broad way about the client's resources, and the client responds.
4. The therapist asks about resources using implicit spiritual language, and the client responds.
5. The therapist asks specifically about the client's spiritual or religious life, and the client responds.

I'll talk about all these beginnings in a moment, but first I'd like to note that I usually proceed in exactly this order. First, I listen to see if the client introduces something explicitly or implicitly spiritual (1 and 2 above). Next, I listen for explicit or implicit spiritual resources, in response to my questions (3 and 4 above). Finally, when necessary, I ask directly about the client's spiritual or religious life (5 above).

I prefer this sequence because I believe that the most helpful clinical interactions happen when spirituality emerges naturally in the flow of a conversation—in the metaphors clients use, the stories they tell, the beliefs they express—more than when I ask about it directly. It also reduces the chance that my particular way of asking will inhibit what clients experience, what they choose to share, and the way they share it.

If clients have a spiritual life, and if they feel safe, they will usually bring it up. We may have to listen carefully to hear it—they may just drop a hint of it as a test to see if it's an OK thing to talk about with us—and when we hear it we need to respond to it. (Otherwise we're not having a conversation; the client is just delivering a monologue.) But clients almost always bring it up, and I rarely have to ask directly and explicitly if spirituality is important to them.

Spiritual conversation, like all conversation, is art and not science. It unfolds in different ways at different times, depending on various cues we're picking up from the client and on our state of mind on a given day. But in general, here is the sequence I follow in making space for spiritual conversation to begin.

The Client Says Something Explicitly Spiritual

The simplest way spiritual conversation begins in therapy is when your client says something that is clearly, unmistakably spiritual:

"I've been meditating and I still feel anxious."
"I wonder if God is punishing me."
"My rabbi thinks I should definitely take the job."
"Since all this happened, I haven't been able to pray."

And there you go. You didn't lift a finger. You didn't egregiously or subtly impose your own spirituality. But lo and behold, a spiritual conversation has begun. We don't know yet how important this spiritual matter is to the client, whether she wants to talk about it a whole lot more, or whether, maybe, we've just been handed the key to her therapeutic universe. But spirituality is now in the room, and the next move is ours, to extend the conversation and see what happens.

There are a thousand ways to keep the conversation going, but I recommend taking it easy. Just say back some short phrase or question that invites the client to say more if she wants. For instance,

Client:	"I've been meditating and I still feel anxious."
Therapist:	"Oh. You meditate. Will you tell me more about that?"
Client:	"I wonder if God is punishing me."
Therapist:	"How do you mean?"
Client:	"My rabbi thinks I should definitely take the job."
Therapist:	"You've talked with your rabbi about this."
Client:	"Since all this happened, I haven't been able to pray."

Therapist: "Not being able to pray—how's that affecting you?"

I've heard Ken Pargament say, "Therapy is not rocket science." And it's true. Brilliance is not required, and if you do happen to be brilliant, it tends to get in the way. The best responses are those that keep the conversation going with minimal intrusiveness. Anyone could say them. That's why the most important question in spiritually integrated psychotherapy is the simplest: "Will you tell me more about that?"

So the client initiates, and the therapist responds. But what happens if the therapist *doesn't* respond?

One possibility is that the client decides spirituality is not a welcome topic of conversation in therapy, or that this spiritual part of herself isn't important or relevant. I've had many clients—and you probably have too—who say about a previous experience in therapy, "I brought this up, and the therapist looked at me like I was crazy."

If you're reading this book, it's clear you don't want this to happen to your clients. So you're going to respond—usually. There are several reasons why you might not. Maybe you just didn't hear it. Your client was mumbling, your mind was wandering, or the lawnmower outside got really loud at exactly the wrong moment.

Maybe you heard what your client said but didn't recognize it as spiritual. She said something using language familiar to people inside her spiritual community but not to you, an outsider. For example, if she said the phrase "right action," and if you're familiar with Buddhism, you'll recognize right action as part of the Eightfold Path and, thus, as a spiritual comment. But if you're not familiar with Buddhism, you might not have noticed.

Or maybe you heard it and recognized it, but you made a clinical decision to go in a different direction in this moment.

Client: "I've been meditating and I still feel anxious."
Therapist: "Would you tell me more about the anxious
            feeling?"

Or maybe you had a countertransference reaction to what the client said, and consciously or unconsciously you decided you can't engage that particular spiritual conversation right now.

All this to say: there are times when a client begins a spiritual conversation and we don't follow up on it. But by and large, if we want to include spirituality in the work we do as therapists, we respond. We make enough contact with the client's comment that, at a minimum, he learns that spirituality is a welcome topic, and even more, we help launch a conversation that proves to be of therapeutic value.

The Client Says Something Implicitly Spiritual

Another way spiritual conversation begins is when the client says something implicitly spiritual. We talked about implicit spiritual experiences in chapter 4. These are experiences of spiritual significance that don't show up wearing a "spirituality" name tag. They include the psychospiritual experiences mentioned in the last chapter, things like gratitude, kindness, despair, and anxiety. When a client uses any of these words or describes an experience to which any of these words might apply, they have possibly begun a spiritual conversation. And so we respond.

Remember what we said earlier. The best responses are simple ones. If a client makes the psychospiritual statement "The things that happened to me then have been a burden ever since," we might ask one of the following questions:

- How do you mean "burden"?
- Can you tell me more about it?

- How is it affecting you?
- Is the burden something you can feel physically?
- Are there thoughts that are part of the burden?
- Are there emotions that are part of it?
- Are there times you feel it more? Times you feel it less?
- Are you feeling it right now, while we're talking about it?

Any of these responses might help a client deepen his connection with this "burden" and allow any possible spiritual undercurrents to surface. Even if this client's burden seems to have no spiritual undercurrents, our response can still deepen our understanding of him and strengthen our connection.

Therapists sometimes feel uneasy when conversations turn toward the spiritual. I've heard many therapists say, "I'm not spiritual enough to work with spirituality," and "I don't know enough to answer the spiritual questions people have." But notice that the menu of responses above are question-based rather than answer-based. They invite collaboration and dialogue, and they don't require you to be a spirituality expert.

Here is a longer example of a client introducing implicit spiritual themes into the therapy process. This example is more complicated, because those themes were introduced in the midst of a crisis. I wanted to make contact with the spiritual themes, which ended up being very important to the therapy, but I wanted to do so briefly, to keep attention where it was needed most at that point, on the crisis.

A successful professional woman, married with two children, has a brief affair with a coworker. She ends the affair without her husband ever knowing. A few months later, her husband plans a special day just for her. It's not her birthday, or their anniversary, or Valentine's Day. He's just living out his love for her. In the midst of that day, she is overcome by the burden of her secret. She breaks down and tells her husband about the affair. He is shocked, hurt, and angry. Five days later they come for their first appointment. Near the end of that appointment, she says, tearfully,

> I feel so bad. So bad for him. It's making me sick. I can't eat. I can't sleep. I can't go to work. I can't do anything to make this up to him. I can't do anything but cry and feel sick. All the good things in my life, I don't deserve any of it. I haven't had to work that hard for any of it. I haven't earned it. There are all these great things in my life, and I'm not worthy of any of it.

This woman's words are full of implicit spiritual themes. We hear guilt, shame, and a sense of unworthiness. We hear the desire to make amends, the longing for atonement and restoration. We hear that she has made confession and begun a season of penitence where she cuts herself off from rest, nourishment, and the fulfillment she experiences through work. We might be hearing, not in her words but in the larger story of the affair, the description of a self not fully integrated, of some important part of herself having been split off, acted out, and now agonizingly dragged into the light, where it might be explored and incorporated into her larger self.

We don't know if guilt, shame, penitence, and the like are spiritual issues in her eyes, and we wouldn't say, "I hear your guilt, shame, and penitence as spiritual issues." We would use the ambiguous psychospiritual language she has introduced and see what unfolds as the client's statement expands into a conversation.

Additionally, in this first appointment after disclosure of an affair, we probably wouldn't move to deepen any of these spiritual themes and explore them fully, unless we had reason to think that deepening one of these themes would help with stabilization. But since we want to let our client know we're listening to things that might be of spiritual significance for her, we would try our best to contact those themes and tag them for later exploration. So in addition to expressing deep empathy for each person's pain and for their anger, asking each of them what they hoped could happen now, and offering a bit of psycho-education about the path to recovery from an affair, I also said this to her:

> The other thing I want to let you know is that I hear how much guilt and shame you're feeling. It's a lot, and it's intense, and it's actually making you sick—physically sick. We won't go deep into those feelings today, but I want you to know I hear them, and they're both really normal and really important. It really hurts to be feeling this way, but if we can support you the right way, they might help take you somewhere good. So it'll probably help if we come back to them and let you feel them and hear what they're saying and how they might be able to help you all through this. Would that be OK?

There are numerous assumptions of theory and technique embedded in that short statement, unrelated to the spirituality focus of this book. My point here is this: listen for the implicitly spiritual statements your clients make and respond to them.[2] Your clients might not even be aware that what they're expressing has a spiritual dimension to it until you slow them down and help them explore it. But your deep hearing and mirroring help open a door.

The Therapist Asks in a Broad Way about the Client's Resources

The next two spiritual conversation starters begin with you, the therapist, asking your client about strengths and resources. In both these next two approaches, we are still not asking explicitly about spirituality. But we are creating space in which clients can tell us something spiritual about themselves, in their own way, on their own terms.

All clients have internal and external resources they draw upon to get through hard times and, beyond just getting through, to feel good and flourish. For many people, at least some of these resources are spiritual in nature. So questions like, "What are some of your strengths?" and "What's been getting you through?" are, in effect, invitations for people to tell us something about themselves spiritually.

We listen for resources and ask questions about resources throughout the course of therapy, but we certainly do that in a first appointment. Let's talk about resource questions in that initial therapeutic encounter.

Probably like most of you, I'm trying to do three things in a first appointment:

1. Make emotional connection with the client.
2. Assess what's going on.
3. Establish some initial therapeutic contract.

That's Connect-Assess-Contract—CAC, if you like acronyms. We can't always accomplish all three in a first meeting, and if I have to choose, I generally prioritize connection over the other two. (The exception, for me, would be a crisis that needs tending immediately, such as a client who is suicidal. In crisis situations, I'll make interventions for safety even if I mess up the connection.)

As part of Connect-Assess-Contract, the bare bones of what I want to learn are as follows:

•   What's going on (the presenting issue, *DSM* symptoms, a bit of context)?
•   How it's affecting them (externally and internally)?

- *What they're doing to try to deal with it* (and how well those things are working)?
- What their theory is about why it's happening (how the client understands or conceptualizes the problem)?
- What they're wanting to happen now (goals)?
- How they feel talking with me about this?

Usually we have to ask about some of these items directly, but since these are things that just make sense to tell someone when you're seeking their help, most clients offer some of this information without our having to ask.

The item I emphasized above, *what they're doing to try to deal with it*, is the part where we're learning about their resources. It often helps to ask broad questions, such as, "What's been getting you through this?" "How have you been surviving in all this?" "What—or whom—are you drawing on for help?"

These questions are not explicitly spiritual, and we may or may not hear spiritual answers. But whatever we learn here will be clinically useful. We'll end up knowing some of our clients' *internal resources*, attributes like intelligence, determination, and a sense of humor. And we'll also find out some of their *external resources*, things outside themselves, like friends, health insurance, and a public park where they like to walk.

Often, even when we're not asking explicitly spiritual questions, what clients tell us about are some of their spiritual resources. "What's been getting you through this?" we might ask. And a client might say, "my meditation practice" or "my friends from church." And here you are, at the trailhead of a spiritual conversation.

We'll talk more about spiritual resources throughout the rest of the book. But here I'll remind you that we're listening not just for explicit spiritual resources (like a meditation practice or friends from church) but also for implicit spiritual resources (like a sense of hope or having neighbors they trust). Here's a table to illustrate the kinds of things we might hear, divided into categories of implicit/explicit and internal/external:

**Explicit and Implicit Spiritual Resources:
Internal and External**

	Explicit Spiritual Resources	Implicit Spiritual Resources
Internal Resources	Sense of connection with God Beliefs Meditation practice	Feeling of purpose Hope Patience
External Resources	Rabbi, Pastor, Imam Sacred site (church, labyrinth) Meditation group	Close friends or family Book group Running club

Again, we'll talk more about spiritual resources in successive chapters—how to evaluate their efficacy and help clients make therapeutic use of them—but for now, just recognize that your curiosity about resources opens space for your clients to introduce spirituality into the therapeutic conversation.

And as we have mentioned already, whatever our clients tell us deserves a response: "Will you tell me more about that?" "How do you mean?" "How does this affect your life?"

The Therapist Asks about Resources Using Psychospiritual Language

This next approach to getting a spiritual conversation started is almost identical to the one we just discussed. What's similar is that we ask about resources without using explicitly spiritual language. What's different is that we load our questions with a bit of psychospiritual language, thus priming[3] clients a teensy bit to consider their psychospiritual resources.

So instead of asking, "What's been getting you through?" we might ask, "What's been sustaining you?" It's a subtle difference, but the word "sustain" has more spiritual resonance than the phrase "getting you through" does.

Here are some other resource questions phrased in more of a psychospiritual vein:

- Where are you drawing strength from?
- Where do you find peace?
- Where do you find hope?
- Is there anybody who truly understands your situation?[4]

Words like *strength*, *peace*, and *hope*, and the idea of someone who truly understands, often have spiritual meaning for people. When we use those words, it's like offering mild electrical stimulation to our clients' spiritual selves, and whatever spiritual feeling they carry around those words will often declare itself.

The Therapist Asks Specifically about the Client's Spirituality or Religion

Thus far, I have described ways spiritual conversation begins in therapy with no prompting from the therapist (the client says something explicitly or implicitly spiritual, and the therapist responds) and with *minimal* prompting (the therapist asks about resources). I have expressed that it's my preference for spiritual conversation to begin in one of these ways, because they serve to keep my own spiritual biases at bay just a little more, leaving space for the client to set the spiritual frame without too much of my meddling. I have also noted that in this approach, especially with spiritual ears attuned to implicit spirituality and psychospiritual language, I almost always find myself involved in spiritual conversation with my client.

That said, sometimes it is helpful to ask directly about spirituality or religion. This might be as follow-up to a spiritual conversation that has begun implicitly, so that I know whether whatever psychospiritual matter we're talking about is connected with some explicit sense of spirituality in the client's mind. Let's say, for example, that I ask a client what's been getting him through this hard time, and he tells me about walking in the woods early in the mornings. I then ask him to tell me more about that, and he says it brings him a sense of peace, that he feels affected by the stillness and strength of the trees. As he goes through the rest of his day, he says, particularly when he's facing the problem that's brought him to therapy, he sees the trees in his mind; tries to be still and strong, like trees are; and imagines breathing like trees breathe, through their skin. If I then wanted to learn whether he feels any explicit spiritual connection to this practice, I might ask, "Those early-morning walks among the trees, and the way you carry that with you during the day, does that have a spiritual feel or some spiritual meaning for you?"

Another time I ask directly about spirituality is near the end of an initial appointment, when I'm doing a quick tour of areas of a client's life we might not have talked about yet.

"We've got just a few minutes left. There are a few things I want to ask you about briefly, and we can come back and talk more about any of them later, but I'd like to run through those with you real quick. That OK?"

"Sure."

And then I ask directly about spirituality and religion, but mixed in with other questions, like these:

- Are you dealing with any health issues we've not talked about yet?
- Are you taking any medications?
- Do you use any illegal drugs or legal drugs that weren't prescribed for you?
- Do you drink alcohol? About how many drinks a week?
- Do you use caffeine? About how much? Nicotine?
- Are you able to exercise? What do you do? How often?
- How satisfying, or not, is the work you do?
- Do you see yourself as a spiritual or religious person?[5]

- Are you connected with a religious community? If so, which one?
- Has your problem affected you religiously or spiritually? If so, in what way?
- Has religion or spirituality been part of how you've been coping with your problem?
- What are the things you do for fun or for self-care?
- The place where you live, do you feel safe there?
- Do you have friends in your life like you want?
- Have there been any major losses in your life? Recently? Or some time ago but they're still affecting you?

In asking directly about spirituality and religion, I'm trying to express to clients that I consider these matters potentially important in their lives and in the work we might do in therapy. By including spirituality and religion alongside some of these other topics, and thus not elevating them above the others, I am trying to keep the playing field level and unbiased. Spirituality is *one* of the things I'm curious about, but not the only thing.

I ask as many of those questions as I can in a first session. But there's usually not enough time for all of them, so I'll work them into the second session. And of course, there's not enough time in a first session to go into depth on any of these topics. What we're doing here, in this quick run-through of important things to know about our client, is putting check marks beside things we will return to and explore in more depth at a later session.

But, with respect to the point of this chapter, a spiritual conversation has begun.

CONCLUSION

I've intentionally saved a word for the very end of this chapter. That word is "collaborative." Being collaborative is important in all aspects of psychotherapy, but in the approach I've described for beginning spiritual conversations in therapy, it's the secret sauce. If we begin with safety, curiosity, openness, and respect; if our spiritual ears are open to the breadth of what's spiritual; and if we respond to what we hear, our clients will almost always lead us into spiritual conversation. The conversation might be implicitly or explicitly spiritual, but a spiritual conversation will have begun.

We don't know where that conversation will go, of course, and the next step in the process is to learn more about who our client is spiritually. Here we come to the topic of the next chapter: spiritual assessment.

6

Spiritual Assessment

What We Need to Know
and How We Come to Know It

A SPIRITUAL CONVERSATION HAS BEGUN. AT MINIMUM, WE know if our client sees herself as spiritual or religious or not. We might also know some of her spiritual resources.

But now we want to go deeper. The heart of therapy is interventions.[1] And before we can intervene in effective and ethical ways, we first need to learn more about who our client is, spiritually and otherwise. We need to know if our client's spirituality is helping him or hurting him. And we need to decide what role, if any, spirituality will play in the therapy. We call this process "spiritual assessment."

There are lots of ways to do spiritual assessment. We can spend weeks and weeks doing a thorough spiritual assessment, but by then our client is probably going to be someone else's client. The approach I'm sharing with you tries to balance learning as much as we can with not overdoing it. The people

I teach tell me they find this approach helpful but not over-whelming—for them or for their clients.[2]

Let me say three things more before we get rolling. First, there are some written assessment instruments, and I don't use any of them. Some clinicians find these helpful, and I've listed a few of them in this endnote if you're interested.[3] But I prefer a conversational approach, learning what I need to know within the flow of a conversation. Spirituality is a relational thing, psychotherapy is a relational thing, and it makes sense to learn about a relational thing in a relational way.

Second, spiritual assessment includes explicit and implicit spirituality. We can conduct a spiritual assessment with a client without either of us ever using an explicitly spiritual word.

And third, spiritual assessment is ongoing, like all the other kinds of assessment we do in psychotherapy. We're always learning more about who our client is spiritually—and who our client is spiritually is always changing, hopefully in ways that are helpful.

SPIRITUAL ASSESSMENT IN SEVEN STEPS

There are lots and lots of things that are interesting and potentially useful to know about our clients spiritually. But for teaching purposes, I've identified seven I think are most important. Sometimes we have to ask directly to learn these things, and sometimes clients tell us without our having to ask. We don't usually learn them in a linear way, in the order I've listed them, just like we don't usually learn the symptoms of depression our client is experiencing in the order they're listed in the *DSM*. But get these seven things in your head, just as you know the nine criteria for depression, and you'll have a roadmap of what to listen for and ask about:

1. Do your clients consider themselves spiritual or religious?

2. What "tribe(s)" are they in?
3. What are their spiritual resources?
4. What is their spiritual personality?
5. What are their spiritual struggles?
6. Is their spirituality helping them or hurting them?
7. Do they want to talk about spiritual issues in therapy?

Now let's talk about each of these seven areas and how we learn about them.

Spiritual or Religious? Or Not?

As I discussed in chapter 4, I believe everyone is spiritual. But what about our clients? Do they consider themselves spiritual in some way? There are simple ways to find out, as we covered in the previous chapter: listening for what the client says without any of our prompting, asking about resources, or asking the direct question "Do you see yourself as spiritual or religious?"

What Tribe(s) Are They In?

If clients do see themselves as spiritual or religious, where is it that they belong? With what group of people do they identify? Or from what group do they see themselves differentiating?

Are they part of a traditional religious community, like a church, synagogue, mosque, or sangha? What is it like? What are its beliefs and practices? How connected is the client to this community? Does she have significant relationships with a minister and strong friendships within the community? Or is she connected only peripherally? Does she go to services or engage other practices (meditation, prayer, study, service, etc.) because she wants to? Or does she do these things from a sense of obligation? Is it the same community she grew up in or a different one? And what's the story of her leaving or staying?

If it's a traditionally religious tribe, what language does it speak, and what are its words for the deity? Vishnu, Shiva,

God, Jesus, Allah, Higher Power, the Universe? It's especially important in therapy to know the spiritual language our clients use to make sense of their experience. As much as possible, that's the language we want to use with them too.

If a client is not part of a traditional religious community, is he part of some implicit spiritual community that is a source of belonging and meaning? These can be groups of people gathered around art, activism, sports, or some other shared passion.

With many clients, this information lands in our laps because the client volunteers it. Spirituality is such an integrated part of their lives, like salt in the ocean, that it shows up frequently in the things they say.

But if it does not, we can ask directly about explicit religious affiliation: "Are you connected with a religious community or a spiritual community? If so, which one?" We can also ask directly about implicit spiritual affiliation: "Is there someplace you feel like you really belong?" "Is there some group you're a part of that makes your heart sing, or that's doing something you feel deeply committed to?"

What Are Their Spiritual Resources?

Remember what we said about resources in the last chapter. A resource is anything that helps us survive or thrive. It can be something external to us—a tree, a dog, a mentor, a group of friends—or something internal—an attribute, a memory, or an insight. Spiritual resources can be explicitly spiritual—the Star of David you wear around your neck, the Fajr you pray before sunrise, the chaplain you talk with at work—or implicitly spiritual—a sense of hope you feel inside, a group you go running with, or a song on the radio that moves you to tears.

People often tell us about their resources without our having to ask:

"I've been praying about this."	An explicit, internal spiritual resource
"I've been talking with my guru about this."	An explicit, external spiritual resource
"My life is a whirlwind right now, but I feel a sense of peace about it."	An implicit, internal resource
"The most joyful part of my week is when I go dancing with my friends."	An implicit, external resource

But if clients don't offer up this information without our prompting, there are questions we can ask. If we don't yet know their spiritual tribe and what spiritual language they speak, it's best to ask these questions using implicit spiritual language. Here are some you might use:

- What's been getting you through this?
- What strengthens you or nurtures you?
- When do you feel most fully alive?
- Where do you find peace?
- What gives you hope?
- What causes you despair?
- Who truly understands your situation?
- When you are afraid or in pain, where do you turn for comfort?
- For what or for whom do you feel deeply grateful?
- To what or to whom are you most devoted?
- To whom or to what do you most freely express love?
- What practices are especially important to you?
- What are some of the "aha!" experiences in your life?
- What gives you a sense of meaning or purpose?
- Why is it important that you are alive?

- What are you striving for in your life?
- How would you like people to remember you when you are gone?[4]

If we do have a sense of our client's spiritual language, any of the questions above can be made more explicitly spiritual. Here are some examples, phrased for a God-talk person:

- How does God connect with you?[5]
- When do you feel connected to God?
- How do you listen for God?
- How do you talk to God?
- What do you imagine God is like?
- What did you learn about God as you were growing up?
- How has your relationship with God changed since then?
- Have there been times you felt especially close to God?
- Have there been times you felt especially cut off from God?
- Are there ever times when you experience a different side of God?
- What do you think God wants for you?
- What do you think God wants from you?[6]

You won't ask all these questions, obviously. You'll pick and choose, depending on what your clients are telling you about, the way they're telling it, and what you already know about them spiritually. And whatever your client tells you, you'll respond with a "tell me more," and you'll continue to learn.

I encourage students and supervisees to read through these questions once a week, for as long as it takes to internalize them. And I offer the same to you. The more you read them, the more they'll pop into your mind at just the right moment in your clinical practice.

What Is Their Spiritual Personality?

Therapists use any number of personality inventories to understand clients and inform the way we work with them: the Myers-Briggs, the Enneagram, not to mention the classic psychoanalytic classifications.

I am not aware of any widely accepted resource on spiritual personality, and I am not trying to create one here. But I do think it's helpful to consider our clients' spiritual personalities, and here are some questions I carry in mind as I get to know clients spiritually:

- Is it easy for them to trust? Or are they more cautious and skeptical?
- Do they come alive spiritually more in groups? Or in solitude?
- Are they spiritual explorers ? Or spiritual homebodies?
- Do they feel safe with God? Or afraid of God?
- Do they feel connected and close to God? Or disconnected and distant?
- Do they connect with God and their spiritual selves more through their head, their heart, or their body?
- Do they connect with God and their spiritual selves more through action and service? Or through contemplative practices?
- How do they relate to spiritual authority? Do they like having a spiritual teacher or guide? Or do they like going it alone?

These surely are not the only things to consider when assessing someone's spiritual personality. I hope you will add to the list.

As I have said, we can learn a lot about our clients' spiritual personalities just by listening. We can also learn by asking any of those questions I've listed above, or by asking any of the resource-related questions listed in the previous section. I am not recommending that you conduct an intense inquiry that helps you put your client in a spiritual personality box from which he can never escape, only that you listen your way to some working hypothesis about how your client tends to engage spiritual experience.

What Are Their Spiritual Struggles?

Another important part of knowing who your client is spiritually is knowing that person's spiritual struggles.

Sometimes a mental health issue or life stressor can lead to a spiritual struggle: a man who is depressed can't get out of bed to attend Saturday sits at the Zen Center; a woman is having conflict with her son and has begun to hate him, and the hate makes her feel cut off from God; a man is having an affair and feels immense guilt—and now that everyone at his synagogue knows, he feels too ashamed to be part of his spiritual community.

Other times the difficulty that someone brings to psychotherapy *is* an actual spiritual struggle. These can be explicit spiritual struggles: after a series of senseless losses, a woman has lost hope and is questioning her faith; a man feels attracted to other men but believes it's a sin to act on those feelings; a woman believes God is punishing her for an abortion she had ten years ago; a man grew up in a church where there was lots of yelling, and he lives in fear of making God angry.

They can also be implicit spiritual struggles:

- How can I get over this guilt and make amends?
- How can I be free from the grip of this addiction?
- What can I do with my life that feels like it matters?
- How can I trust others enough to be vulnerable with them?

- Why do I exhaust myself doing things for others and neglect myself?
- How will I ever make sense of this suffering?
- How do I turn off this constant chatter in my mind and find a little peace?

As with other parts of their spiritual lives, clients will often name their spiritual struggles without our having to ask. But if they do need a nudge, we can ask implicit spiritual questions like these:

- What are the deepest questions your situation has raised for you?
- How has this experience changed you at the deepest levels?
- What are your deepest regrets?
- What would you like to be able to let go of in your life?

Or explicit spiritual questions like these:

- Has your problem affected you religiously or spiritually? If so, in what way?[7]
- How has your relationship with God affected how you approach this difficulty?
- How has this difficulty affected your relationship with God?

We'll talk more about spiritual struggles in chapter 8.

Is Their Spirituality Helping Them or Hurting Them?

Spirituality can be a force for good and for evil. This is true on a historical scale: human history is replete with religiously motivated goodness and religiously motivated evil. It's also true on a personal scale. Sometimes spiritual beliefs, values, and practices are helping our clients. Sometimes they're hurting. And sometimes it's an ambiguous mix of both. Part of assessment involves asking ourselves how people's spiritual experiences are affecting them: for good or for ill?

This question—Is spirituality helping or hurting my client?—makes many therapists uncomfortable. "Who am I to judge?" we ask. "Am I not imposing my own values and beliefs if I answer that question?"

This is a healthy pause, I think, and a mark of ethical integrity and spiritual humility. Our own spiritual histories and spiritual perspectives affect the way we view other people's spirituality, and we all have different understandings of what healthy looks like. But if we're working with spirituality in psychotherapy, we can't ignore this part of spiritual assessment.

Imagine, for example, a client in a physically, emotionally, or sexually abusive marriage who feels unable to leave because of a religious prohibition.

Or a parent who abuses his children, physically or emotionally, and gives spiritual reasons to justify the abuse: "Spare the rod, spoil the child," which is not in the Bible, and "Children, obey your parents," which is.

Or a man who suffered a traumatic assault and is experiencing symptoms of PTSD but doesn't want to talk about what happened because he's put it in God's hands and is trusting God to heal him.

Or a woman who is chronically depressed. Her depression and meditation practice have commingled in such a way for her that "letting go of thoughts" becomes a way of dissociating from painful matters that are nonetheless important. (Buddhist psychotherapist John Welwood calls this "spiritual bypass."[8])

As much as we don't want to judge other people's spirituality, there are times we must make a clinical decision about whether our clients' spiritual beliefs and practices are helping or hurting them.

Fortunately, we have some help. James Griffith is a psychiatrist working in a cross-cultural setting, often with political refugees, and he has written two incredibly helpful books about the complex relationship between spirituality and mental health issues: *Religion That Heals, Religion That Harms* and *Encountering the Sacred in Psychotherapy*, coauthored with Melissa Elliott Griffith.

In *Encountering the Sacred in Psychotherapy*, Griffith and Griffith say that spiritual beliefs, practice, and communities are healthy when they "point to solutions for life's problems, when they provide meaning, when they engender communion with others, and when their real effects on self and others move toward justice." They are harmful "when they obscure solutions, when they foster despair, or when they isolate people or generate animosity among them."[9]

Notice that the emphasis is on assessing the *impact* that spirituality has on the client's life, not the *truth-claims* of the client's spiritual beliefs. As therapists, we do not engage in philosophical or theological debate with our clients. That is a recipe for activating our clients' defenses and slowing the process of change. We are making assessment, as best we can, about whether their spiritual beliefs and practices help them sustain postures of hope, purpose, meaning, coherence, agency, and the like, and whether their beliefs and practices help them to be more compassionate and moral persons.

We'll talk more harmful spirituality in chapter 9—how to spot it and what to do about it. For now, though, the point is a simple one: assess it.

Do They Want to Talk about Spiritual Issues in Therapy?

The way our clients have already talked about spiritual issues, or not, has given us a pretty good idea about whether it's an important part of their life, whether they see it playing a part in their difficulties or their recovery, and whether they feel comfortable talking with us about it. Even so, it's always good to ask, "Do you want to talk about any of this with me?" Sometimes we'll be surprised by a yes when we were expecting no, or a no when we were expecting yes.

CONCLUSION

I've given you seven basic questions to carry in your head as you talk with your client. You might learn answers to all seven questions in the first few sessions, or you might gather bits and pieces over a longer period of time. You'll also learn things about your client spiritually that don't fit into any of those seven boxes. But when you can answer those seven questions, you've done a pretty good spiritual assessment.

Remember that the point of spiritual assessment is not for us to decide what's right about someone's spirituality and what isn't, or to tell them what's good for them and what's not. The point is to understand who our client is spiritually, to know how to speak their language, to identify resources that might help them, to listen for stuck places or harmful dynamics, and to make decisions about when, where, and how we might intervene.

Spiritual intervention is the subject of the next three chapters. Read on!

7

....

Working with
Spiritual Resources

Spiritual Interventions, Part 1

YOU'VE DONE AN ASSESSMENT. YOU UNDERSTAND YOUR CLI-
ent's presenting issue, related stressors and struggles, and the
impact these things are having on her. You know how she'd
like things to be different and what she's tried already to make
that happen. You know some of what she regards as resources,
spiritual and otherwise, and you've begun hypothesizing about
how to mobilize these resources or connect her with additional
resources to help her feel better and have more of what she
really wants. Now you're ready to act on your hypotheses, to
say something or do something to benefit your client. You're
ready to use an intervention.

Interventions are the reason people come to therapy. Your
client could have continued to ponder her problem in solitude,
or talk about it with the friends and family with whom she's

been discussing it. But she wants additional help, and she's come to you.

Interventions are any of those things you do, verbally or nonverbally, to bring about one of the following outcomes:

- Help clients move toward one of their stated goals.
- Help clients build the stronger foundation they'll need *before* they can move toward one of their stated goals.[1]
- Strengthen the therapeutic alliance.
- Strengthen clients' motivation for change.

Spiritual interventions are any of those things you do, verbally or nonverbally, to help your clients use spiritual resources or engage a spiritual issue for any of those same reasons.

There are hundreds of spiritual interventions, and almost as many ways to organize and classify them. I cannot describe every possible spiritual intervention you might use to help your client. I can only give you a sampling. Nor can I gather these samplings into a single orderly system. I can organize them only loosely, under a few overlapping groupings. And I cannot convey exactly which intervention you should use in a given clinical moment and how *you* would say it or do it. Spiritual interventions, like all other therapeutic interventions, are a bit of an art form, offered in a style and with a sense of timing unique to each therapist and suitable for a particular moment in the course of therapy. There are a thousand ways to do it right.

What I can convey, however, though it's just a drop in the bucket, is still very much worth conveying. I can share with you *some* spiritual interventions, *some* ways to organize them in your own mind, and *some* illustrations. And in all of this, I can suggest to you both the great range of spiritual interventions and the collaborative spirit in which to offer them most effectively.

In this chapter, I will talk about interventions that make use of healthy spiritual resources. In chapter 8 I'll discuss interventions with spiritual struggles. And in chapter 9 I'll describe how to intervene when we believe our client's spirituality is causing harm.

Let me say two more things before we dive in, and these are the two most important things. First, *an intervention is an experiment.* We never know for sure if it's going to help our client or not. And we can't know until we try it and see what happens. If it helps, great! If not, also great! Now we know and can try something different. So, don't be like a dog with a bone and keep pushing an intervention on your client that is not a fit for him. And don't feel discouraged either. It was just an experiment.

That said, here's the equally most important thing: *a good intervention is based on assessment.* Just because interventions are experiments doesn't mean we offer them randomly and indiscriminately. The intervention we choose as an experiment is an extension of the assessment we've done.

WORKING WITH SPIRITUAL RESOURCES

An intervention is an experiment based on assessment. And part of what you've assessed is your client's spiritual resources. Thus, you know, for instance, that your client sings hymns silently to himself throughout the day (an internal spiritual resource) and that he talks regularly with his AA sponsor (an external spiritual resource). Or you know that she reads the Bible each morning (an explicit spiritual resource) while sitting quietly by the window drinking a cup of coffee (an implicit spiritual resource).

I think of there being three kinds of resource-focused spiritual interventions:

1. Strengthening an existing spiritual resource
2. Reconnecting with a forgotten spiritual resource
3. Opening space for a new spiritual resource

I'll now describe and illustrate each of these.

Strengthening an Existing Spiritual Resource

Our client is doing something that's helping. He's listening to a special playlist in the car each morning, or meditating on a passage of Scripture that's become meaningful to him, or talking to his minister several times a week. Let's see if we can strengthen or deepen his connection with that already-established resource and find out what happens.

The simplest way to strengthen an existing resource is to ask the client to tell you more about it. By calling attention to the resource and inviting the client to elaborate on it, you are amplifying the impact that resource has in the client's life. Here's an example:

Therapist: What's been getting you through all this?" *[Here we're doing spiritual assessment.]*[2]

Client: I've been saying this mantra to myself, over and over: "We're all bigger than our mistakes." *[Here the client tells us about an internal, implicit spiritual resource.]*

Therapist: Oh, wow. I love that line. Will you tell me more about it? *[Here is our intervention, to strengthen the client's connection with this resource.]*

Client: It's something my eighth-grade teacher told me once, when I got in trouble for cheating in his class. I got a zero on the test, I had in-school suspension, they called my parents, and I was completely ashamed. He could tell, I know. And he said something to me about how what I'd done was wrong and he hoped I would learn from it, and then he said, "We're all bigger than our mistakes." And obviously, I need to hear that now. A lot.

I've said earlier that the most important question in spiritually integrated psychotherapy is a simple one—"Will you tell me more about that?"—and here we see that question in action, as an intervention to strengthen an existing spiritual resource.

A slightly more sophisticated way of strengthening an existing resource is to help clients experience that resource across as many of the five building blocks of experience as possible. Pat Ogden, chief developer of Sensorimotor Psychotherapy, describes these as "thoughts (cognitions), emotions, perceptions (internally generated images, tastes, smells, touch, and sounds), body movements, and body sensations."[3] All human experience comprises these five elements, and we can help deepen a person's spiritual resource by inviting her to expand her awareness to as many of these five elements as possible.

Therapist: I can tell this phrase means a lot to you, and it's helping you: "We're all bigger than our mistakes." *[This resource is a thought, organized around cognition.]* I'm wondering, when you say those words to yourself, what else do you notice? Is there a feeling that comes with that? Or do you notice anything happening in your body?

Client: Um . . . I actually feel a lot of emotion. [His voice gets raspy.)] I don't know what it is. It's kinda like sadness. But mainly it's just emotion.

Therapist: Yeah, just stay with that. . . . Let it happen. . . . [Client gets a withdrawn expression on his face. He drops his head, curls his shoulders, and leans forward slightly.] And maybe notice where you feel it physically.

Client: [He passes his hand in front of his chest, in a circle, and then in front of his face, also in a circle.] All in here.

Therapist: OK. Just let that happen. [Silence. After a minute, client sits up taller and lifts his face.] And what are you noticing now?

Client: It was kind of like . . . I had a flush of shame, and
               then that finished, and then I actually felt the
               impact of those words in a deeper way. I felt some-
               thing release.

Therapist: Yeah, I could see that. You actually got bigger.
               [Here I sit up taller and lift my face, mirroring
               what he had done a moment earlier.]

Client: Whoa.

Therapist: Yeah. Just let that soak in. . . . We're all bigger
               than our mistakes. . . . You are bigger than your
               mistakes.

Reconnecting with a Forgotten Spiritual Resource

There are a number of questions that can help clients reconnect
with a forgotten spiritual resource that has served them in the
past but is presently not available or accessible to them. These
questions can be stated in an explicitly or implicitly spiritual
way. Here are a few examples:

- Was there a time in the past when you felt more connected to God?
- What's sacred for you?
- What do you do that brings you joy [or peace or
  comfort]?
- Is there a person [or place] that brings out the best in
  you?

Consider this example: Wayne is sixty, married, and the
father of three adult children. One of his children, a son, has a
significant mental illness, and Wayne came to therapy shortly
after this son, without any prior history of violence, attacked
Wayne with a knife. This son now lives in a private-pay group
home that takes a good portion of Wayne's income. Wayne

earns a good salary, but his job is quite stressful, he is tired, and he longs for the day when he can retire. He and his wife have not saved enough for retirement, and with the added financial demand of providing for his son, he wonders how he will ever stop working.

Wayne identifies as Christian. His faith has been important to him since early adulthood. He prays daily, reads devotional literature several times a week, and attends church most Sundays.

In this session, Wayne was expressing his weariness and worry. His voice felt heavy, and his body posture was slumped. I was thinking, *There is no magic wand to wave over his circumstances to make them any easier. But are there any spiritual resources that might help him—not change his circumstances, which seem pretty unalterable—but live with them any differently?*

After lots of mirroring and empathy on my part, we had the following exchange:

Russell: I want to ask you three or four questions. Don't worry about answering all of them, or maybe not any of them. But let them land and percolate in you for a bit, and see what happens. Sound OK? *[Here I'm setting up the intervention and asking permission.]*

Wayne: Sure.

Russell: What's something you do, or have done in the past, that brings you a little bit of peace? Or what are you doing, and where are you, when you feel some sense of hope? Or what do you do, or where, that helps you feel more connected to God? *[The intervention is to ask about forgotten spiritual resources. I phrase the questions to make space for implicit or explicit spiritual resources.]*

Wayne: [Pause] I used to sit on the patio behind the house on Sunday afternoons. I'd take a book and listen to music. But mostly just sit there. It was very restorative. Now it's hard to do that. We're going to church again on Sunday mornings, and with everything else I've got to get done on Sundays, I don't feel like I've got time to do both. But maybe I could make time to sit out there some more. *[He describes an implicit spiritual resource: being outside, with music and a book.]* [He pauses a minute before continuing.] I'll tell you something else. This just popped into my head. A couple nights ago I dreamed there were two men at the foot of my bed. One standing, one sitting at the end of the bed. They were looking at me like they were worried about me. It was right at that moment when I was waking up, so it felt kind of like a dream and kind of like it was real.

Russell: Wow. What's that dream mean to you as you think about it right now?

Wayne: I guess . . . I think . . . I guess they're angels. *[Here he is describing an explicit spiritual resource.]* [Another brief pause.] When I was really young, about five, my mom had a nervous breakdown, and they had to put her in the hospital. My dad dropped me off to stay a few weeks with his sister. You know how they're separating kids from their parents at the border, and how they say that's bad for kids?

Russell: Yeah.

Wayne: Well, I can tell you: it is. My aunt was not a good person, and those weeks with her were just horrible. And there were two angels that were with me and protected me from her.

Russell: Wow.

Wayne: And at different times in my life, I've felt like
             angels were watching over me. But I haven't
             thought about that in a long time.

Russell: And then you had this dream, of the men, or
             angels.

Wayne: Maybe they're still with me.

Russell: Yeah, maybe so. And I wonder what it would be
             like if you could sense those angels around you a
             little more. Or imagine them with you from time
             to time. I don't mean get hyperaware and look for
             them in any kind of anxious way. But just to sense
             around you, through the day, and notice if it feels
             like they're with you. *[Here I am trying to deepen
             his connection with this resource.]*

Wayne: I don't know. I'll see. I'll try noticing. But right
             now, just talking about it, I feel so much more
             calm.

Opening Space for a New Spiritual Resource

Sometimes neither a currently utilized spiritual resource
nor some previously experienced resource, remembered and
brought forward into the present, is enough to help clients cope
with their stress or make meaning of their situation. Sometimes
clients need to develop a new spiritual resource. (And sometimes we do, too!)

In these moments, we can use curiosity, humility, and a
bit of wisdom to help clients expand their spiritual repertoire.
Here is an illustration.

Jerry has come to therapy for help with anxiety. He says he
worries a lot, and once a week he gets a headache that lasts all
day. He talks quickly, and sometimes I have to interrupt him to
make a comment or ask a question that feels important. Jerry

is Jewish. He attends synagogue on the High Holy Days, and he says he prays many times a day.

Russell: Could I ask you more about the praying?

Jerry: Sure.

Russell: Like . . . how you do it. How you pray. Whether you say much, what it feels like. Things like that.

Jerry: Um . . . I mean—I call it praying. But if you were in my head listening, it would probably sound like I was just talking to myself.

Russell: It might sound to me like you're talking to yourself, but to you, you feel like you're talking to God.

Jerry: Right.

Russell: Can I ask what kinds of things you say to God, what you ask God?

Jerry: It's mostly saying. I don't think I ask God for anything. . . . That's interesting, isn't it?

Russell: Yes. It is. But how do you mean?

Jerry: I think most people ask God for stuff. I assume that they do. But I don't think about asking God for any kind of help. *[Jerry and I have stumbled upon a feature of his spiritual personality: a tendency to be spiritually self-reliant rather than spiritually dependent. I can now experiment with helping him stretch that aspect of his spiritual personality and open to a new resource.]*

Russell: Yeah. What happens inside you—what do you think or feel or notice in your body—when you even think about that: about asking God for help?

Jerry: I—I—I feel pretty uncomfortable. Like . . . "help" is such a simple word, but I can't imagine what it would feel like to come out of my mouth, or my heart, or whatever.

Russell: Yeah. So I wonder. Would you be open to experimenting with that a little bit?

Jerry: How would I do that?

Russell: Well, maybe just imagine God listening to you, and just notice what happens inside when you let yourself say the word "help." You can say it aloud or silently. There's not a right or wrong, a this should happen or that should happen, or anything. Just say it and see what you notice.

Jerry: [He drops his eyes and is quiet for a moment. Then he lifts his head and looks at me.] I felt really small. Small in a good way.

The conversation continued from there, and for reasons of space I will not continue the report. But what I have offered you illustrates, I hope, the way that the collaborative conversation has opened space for the client to grow into a new spiritual resource: asking for help.

Here is another example, this one involving a spiritual experience the client had never had before and was uncomfortable having.

Jasmine came to therapy grieving the unexpected death of her father four weeks earlier. They were very close, and she felt devastated by the loss. She took two weeks off from work, but she has not been able to make it through a full day since returning to work. She said she doesn't want to get over losing him, but she needs the money from working and wants to be able to hold herself together.

I was asking her what she's been doing to try to hold herself together at work when I felt a shift of energy in the room and noticed her face had become alert and still. I interrupted what I was saying and sat quietly with her for a few moments.

Russell: Did something just happen?

Jasmine: This is very strange, but I can feel him here now.

Russell: Where is he? [She points, with her head, to her right, toward a large plant in front of one of the windows.] Is it OK with you that he's here?

Jasmine: [She nods yes.] This is really weird. I don't believe in stuff like this. [Pause.] But it's OK.

Russell: OK. So is it all right if I make a suggestion? [She nods yes again.] Maybe tell him you're OK with him being here. You can do it silently or aloud, whichever seems like the right way. [I pause and wait on her.] And let me know what happens.

Jasmine: He's just here. Nothing else is happening.

Russell: OK. How about if you ask him how come he's here.

Jasmine: [Silence] He just wants me to know he's still here, he still loves me, he's still with me. [She is silent for a few moments, with a soft look on her face.] This feels so good, in a way, and also so weird. But I'm really glad he's here.

Russell: Yes. That make sense. Just . . . in a soft way, if you can . . . just tell him all that. Let him know this feels a little weird to you but that it also feels good and you're grateful he's come.

Jasmine: [She begins crying gently.] It feels like he's come closer. Not physically closer. He's still over there. But . . . emotionally closer. Closer to my heart.

Russell: So just let that happen. Let him be here with you. Let yourself be with him.

Some therapists are very much at ease with the idea that people can communicate with deceased loved ones or other spiritual beings, and some are not. But either way, some clients have these experiences and will want to know if they can talk with you about them. And sometimes, as in the example above, they might have such an experience in your office.

Several years ago I shared this example with a group I was training, and one person in particular was very uncomfortable hearing about it. "You are freaking me out," she told me. I validated her discomfort, thanked her for sharing it, and we talked about it a lot. Three months later, she reported that a nearly identical encounter happened in her office, with one of her clients. "I just took a deep breath, said to myself, 'OK, let's do it,' and did my best to support the conversation. It was maybe the most powerful session I've ever been part of."

COMMONLY USED SPIRITUAL RESOURCES

In this next section, I mention some of the more commonly used interventions that leverage spiritual resources. All of these have been the subject of considerable research, and their benefits for physical and mental health are widely documented. My treatments of these interventions will be minimal, not because they are unimportant but because much has already been written about them elsewhere. I will refer you, in the endnotes, to resources where you can read and learn more. I begin with interventions that are more implicitly spiritual and proceed to some that are explicitly spiritual.

Mindfulness

"Mindfulness," says Jon Kabat-Zinn, perhaps its most well-known popularizer, "means paying attention in a particular way: on purpose, in the moment and nonjudgmentally."[4]

Mindfulness is surely the most widely used spiritual intervention in psychotherapy. Numerous therapy models are explicit in their use of mindfulness—Dialectical Behavioral Therapy,

Acceptance and Commitment Therapy, Mindfulness-Based Cognitive Behavioral Therapy, Sensorimotor Psychotherapy, Hakomi, Internal Family Systems Therapy, and others—but any therapeutic modality that asks clients to notice what's happening inside is using mindfulness.

Not everyone considers mindfulness a spiritual intervention, of course, and persons can practice (and teach) mindfulness without any explicit spiritual reference. But the roots of mindfulness are in Buddhism, and while he is now careful to avoid any semblance of explicit spiritual language, Jon Kabat-Zinn developed his Mindfulness-Based Stress Reduction (MBSR) trainings after studying with Buddhist teachers like Thich Nhat Hanh. Mindfulness engages human faculties that all religious traditions would claim as spiritual, and the practice at the heart of mindfulness, relating to our experience without judgment, is a highly evolved spiritual capacity.

Therapists can bring mindfulness into sessions in a variety of ways. We can recommend to our clients one of the many good books[5] or podcasts[6] that teach mindfulness, or refer them to an MBSR class.[7] Some more conservative Christian clients have a negative association to the word "mindfulness." But if we've done a spiritual assessment, we will know this and probably not use that word with them.

We can also employ mindfulness in session without ever using the word itself. We might do this when a client is emotionally dysregulated and wants help getting back to a state of emotional regulation. Here we might offer the 4-3-2-1 tool:

- Look slowly around the office, and notice *four* things blue or green.
- Now go inside and notice *three* different physical sensations happening right now in your body.
- Now listen for *two* different sounds.
- Now notice *one* slow, easy breath.

Or we might introduce mindfulness into the flow of a conversation to help a client explore the meaning of a recurring experience, giving directives or asking questions that our client can answer only by paying attention to her right-here-right-now inner experience. When we're integrating mindfulness into a session, we use the word "notice" a lot.

Client: My boss hates me.

Therapist: Yes, you feel that way a lot. And I wonder, could you notice, as you have that thought right now and say it to me—"my boss hates me"—notice what happens inside you right now: what emotions, what sensations in your body, what other thoughts.

Client: I just feel this pit in my stomach, like I'm gonna get fired any day. And how am I gonna survive?

Therapist: Got it: a pit in your stomach, and thoughts about getting fired and how will you make it. . . . So if you can, just stay with that for a moment, that pit in your stomach, that worry. And notice what happens next.

Client: It reminds me of when I was in third grade, and my dad got fired, and we had to move.

Therapist: OK. So go with that a minute, that memory, and notice what happens inside.

Client: I just feel so helpless. Like there's nothing I can do.

The therapist might then pursue some further intervention, perhaps to explore how the client's threatening boss reminds him of that third-grade experience when she was powerless, and how the emotional and somatic residue of that childhood experience is blocking the client's access to her full capacity and strength as an adult. The therapist might then help the client call forward some adult strengths that can serve her more effectively in this difficult situation. Whatever path forward we might take as therapists—and there are a thousand ways to do it right—we got to that point through an intervention that invited the client to slow down and pay attention to her experience.

Meditation

Research on the benefits of meditation is ongoing,[8] but the scientific community is amassing compelling evidence that meditation lowers stress chemicals in the bloodstream, boosts our immune system, lowers blood pressure, and lessens the effects of depression, anxiety, ADHD, and age-related cognitive decline. In some studies, people who meditated just eight weeks showed growth in the areas of the brain related to self-awareness and compassion.

There are many, many ways to meditate, some of them explicitly spiritual, some not. Some approaches to meditation involve focusing our attention: on the breath, a mantra, an icon, or a candle. Some involve no particular focusing at all, simply activating our inner observer and noticing whatever arises in our minds, hearts, and bodies. Others involve letting go of whatever arises, allowing ourselves to empty as completely as possible. I like Teresa of Ávila's description of meditation as "resting in stillness," but we can meditate while walking, running, washing dishes, singing—you name it. The common feature across all forms of meditation is this intention: to be more awake to reality as it is and less a captive of the habits and compulsions of our ordinary state of consciousness.

We want to introduce meditation in a way that is a spiritual fit for our client—and again, only to those clients who do not have some overly negative association to the idea of meditating. There are many excellent books on Christian meditation[9] and Buddhist meditation,[10] and two of my favorite books on meditation are by Muslims.[11] There are also many wonderful resources on meditation for people who are nonreligious or antireligious.[12]

Several of my clients like to begin their sessions with five minutes of silent meditation. I ring a prayer bowl to start and end the period of silence, and something happens for them and me that helps the session be more useful to them. Other times, in the middle of a session, with a client who has identified meditation as a spiritual resource, in a moment when they are seeming stuck or feeling overwhelmed, I might ask them if they'd like to take a pause to meditate.

Guided Imagery

Guided imagery is a variant of meditation. In guided imagery, the therapist uses words to help a client enter an imaginary scene, usually one where the client can feel safe or relaxed, occasionally one in which the client can feel empowered. The therapist typically suggests the broad frame of some scene, then invites the client to detail it using as many of her senses as make sense: sight, sound, touch, smell, and taste. In EMDR (Eye Movement Desensitization and Reprocessing) therapy, for instance, one of the first interventions is a guided imagery intervention, inviting the client to create a safe place.

You can find a gazillion guided imagery scripts online. Just enter "guided imagery script" into your search engine, for scripts that are implicitly spiritual, or "guided imagery Jesus" or "guided imagery Buddha" for scripts that are more explicitly spiritual.

Here is a short guided imagery script, just to give you a taste:

> Allow to come to mind some place where you feel safe,
> or at ease, or happy. It might be a place you've been

before, a place you visit often, or an imaginary place. It can be indoors or outdoors. Take your time.

As this place begins to appear in your mind and heart, allow yourself to look around slowly. Notice what you see there: the colors, the quality of the light, whether you're alone or whether other people are there. Notice where you are, whether you're sitting, standing, lying down, or moving in some way. Notice the temperature, the way the air feels on your skin, what you're touching, or what's touching you. Maybe notice any sounds happening in this place. Notice if there are any smells or tastes that come with being here.

Let yourself just be there, and settle, in whatever way feels right and good to you. And notice the quality of your breath in this place. Notice other sensations in your body.

You might want to give this place a name, or let it give itself a name.

You can stay here a while longer if you'd like. You can leave whenever you're ready, just by slowly opening your eyes. And you can return whenever you need.

This is an implicitly spiritual script. You can also find scripts that are explicitly spiritual, if that is appropriate for your client. And even with this one, the client may experience it in an explicitly spiritual way.

And just in case you're wondering, it's fine for you to ask if your clients are willing to describe their safe place to you. Describing it to you helps deepen it as a resource for them.

Gratitude

Every spiritual tradition I know recognizes the importance of gratitude—"If you give thanks, I will give you more" (Quran

14:7); "O give thanks to the LORD, for he is good" (Psalm 136:1)—and science agrees. Gratitude reduces toxic emotions, elevates mood, increases resilience, improves relationships, increases willpower, and even helps people sleep better.

If you want to learn more about the science and spirituality of gratitude, check out the great work of Robert Emmons. He's a psychologist who has authored several scholarly and popular books about gratitude and conducted a three-year study funded by the Templeton Foundation on the impact of gratitude among Christian teenagers. One of his recommendations is that people keep a gratitude journal, taking a few minutes each day to slow down, call to mind something from the day they're grateful for, savor the details, and write it down.

Altruism

In many of the same ways that gratitude is beneficial for us, so is doing good. Reaching out to others, lending a hand, giving away money, volunteering, smiling at a stranger, picking up trash—any of these actions can improve our overall physical and mental health. Plus, it feels good: acts of service release endorphins in the human body.

Our clients are often inwardly motivated to serve others, and if so, we can affirm that and encourage it. Sometimes, when clients are depressed, disheartened, or at a stuck place in their lives, a suggestion to involve themselves in service can get them back on the road to health. There are exceptions, of course—clients who overdo it, serving others at the price of self-neglect, exhaustion, or burnout—but for many people, the spiritually endorsed prescriptions for kindness, mercy, and justice are good medicine.

Use of Sacred Texts

Many clients find Scripture to be a significant resource in their lives, and incorporating their Scripture into therapy is often helpful. Scott Richards and Allen Bergin are frequently quoted on this topic, and they say that Scripture can be used to help clients "(a) challenge and modify their dysfunctional beliefs; (b) reframe and understand their problems and lives from an eternal, spiritual perspective; (c) clarify and enrich their understanding of the doctrines of their religious tradition; (d) strengthen their sense of spiritual identity and life purpose; and (e) seek God's enlightenment, comfort, and guidance."[13]

Clients often introduce Scripture themselves, with no prompting from us. "I respect my parents because it tells me to in the Quran," someone might tell us. Or "I feel like Jacob wrestling with the angel." Our role in these moments is never to debate or correct our clients about Scripture. It is to bring curiosity to what they share and, if it seems advisable, to help strengthen their connection with this resource. "What does this passage mean to you?" "How do you see yourself in that story?" "What emotion do those words bring up in you?"

Sometimes, though, after our assessment has shown us that a particular Scripture is important in a client's life, we might be the ones who introduce Scripture into a moment of psychotherapy. We do this not with the intention to instruct or advise, but to see if their Scripture might be a forgotten resource that can help them in their current moment. "Is there a verse from the Scripture, or a story, that shines any light on this situation?" "Is there a character from your Scripture whom you relate to in some way?"

Whatever they say, with or without any prompting on our part, our response is, "Tell me more, tell me more."

There are many Scriptures, of course:

- In Hinduism: the Vedas
- In Buddhism: the Tripitaka (Pali Canon)
- In Taoism: the Tao Te Ching
- In Judaism: the Tanakh,[14] the Talmud, and Midrash

- In Christianity: the Bible
- In Islam: the Quran

And sometimes the Scripture that is sacred to our client is one that is also sacred to us. Even so, we should not assume that Scripture means the same thing to our client that it does to us. Our work is to help them draw upon Scripture in a way that works for them, not to bring them into alignment with our way of seeing.

That said, there are times when it will seem to us that our clients are using Scripture in ways that are harmful to them or to someone else, and we will undoubtedly want to do what we can to change this. Here we are in the territory of how to work with harmful spirituality and religion, and I will talk about this in chapter 9.

Prayer

Anne Lamott has a wonderful book about prayer titled *Help, Thanks, Wow*. The name alone expresses much about the reasons people pray: to ask for help, to say thanks, and to express wonder. Some people pray regularly, others occasionally, and some not at all. Some pray with a particular deity in mind, some to their ancestors, some to the Earth itself, or to the Universe. Some pray words they have memorized, some pray their own words, some pray in utter silence. Others pray with their hands, with their feet, or with music.

In all its diverse forms, for all its diverse motivations, prayer is a spiritual resource for many clients. And we can integrate prayer into psychotherapy in a variety of ways.

Most easily, we can suggest prayer as an out-of-session intervention. For clients who report prayer as one of their spiritual resources, we can encourage them to deepen their connection with prayer: to talk with spiritual leaders or friends about prayer, to ask others to pray for them, to pray at regular times of the day, to pray at moments in which they don't usually think about praying, and to explore different ways to pray (writing their prayers, reading prayers others have written, doing more listening than talking, and the like).

We therapists can also pray for our clients: outside of session; silently, in the middle of session; and aloud, in session.

Praying aloud with clients in session is an intervention some therapists are open to using, even enjoy using, and some are not. Either way is fine. But if you do pray aloud with clients, it's important to recognize that this is an intervention in which we are most likely to impose our own spiritual beliefs and practices on our clients, and we should proceed with great care. Several authors have written helpfully on this topic,[15] and if you are considering praying aloud with your clients, or if you already do, I encourage you to read these works and take them to heart.

While you have this book in hand, though, let me offer several thoughts about using in-session, out-loud prayer as an intervention. First, there are many good therapeutic reasons to pray in session with clients. Here are eight, borrowed with some adaptation from the work of Peter Gubi:[16]

1. To build rapport and trust
2. To help with emotional regulation
3. To deepen a client's connection to emotion or somatic experience
4. To deepen a client's capacity for honesty and reduce self-deception
5. To deepen a person's connection to God or his spiritual experience
6. To strengthen a client's capacity to ask for help
7. To validate an already expressed thought or feeling
8. To gently lead a client toward understanding or articulating a previously unrecognized thought or feeling

Can you think of others?

If you do take the prayer plunge, I hope you will keep several thoughts in mind:

Never pray to proselytize. There are honorable professions where proselytization is expected and permissible, e.g., rabbi, pastor, imam, etc. Therapist is not one of them.

Pray aloud only if you have a clear sense of who your client is spiritually, what language they speak, whether prayer is meaningful to them, and how they pray.

Pray aloud only in the language that is native to your client, and only if that language has integrity for you.

Pray aloud only if it is something you can do with authenticity. Only pray in a way that feels real for you (the style of prayer), and only for things you are comfortable praying for (the content of prayer).

If you're not comfortable praying aloud, don't. If your client asks you to pray and you don't want to—not with him, in particular, or not with anyone, ever—just say that prayer is a private practice for you, and not something you want to do aloud. Then ask him how your response lands with him. And offer to listen to his prayer.

Pray aloud only with your client's consent. Sometimes your client might ask you to pray for her or with her. Sometimes you might offer to pray for your client or with her. But never just start praying.

Be very careful about initiating prayer with clients who have trouble setting boundaries or who are prone to please you or follow your every suggestion.

Be careful that praying with you is not creating an easy out for your client. For some clients, prayer is a way to avoid seeking truth and being challenged. Ask yourself if praying with you will weaken the client's resolve to change—by implying that there's an outside fixer who can take care of this issue for the client, just the way the client wants it—without the client having to stretch himself.

Be careful that praying with the client is not creating an easy out for you. Therapists can be tempted to pray when we find it hard to continue listening to our client, when we want to escape the pain or helplessness of being with her and her difficulty, when we want to speed the client through grief or pain, or when we are uncomfortable with her feelings and want to tidy them up. Will offering to pray give us an escape but leave our client feeling abandoned?

Pray aloud only if you have considered how it might affect the transference. Will praying aloud create any subtle pressure for the client to think, feel, or act like you?

Also consider the countertransference. Are you feeling pressured to pray? Will you feel performance anxiety? Are you feeling overexposed and more vulnerable than you want?

Connect with your heart before you speak a word, and whatever you say, keep it short and simple.

SPIRITUAL INTERVENTIONS
IN FOUR DIMENSIONS

There's another way of thinking about spiritual interventions that I call the "four dimensions." It's a way of organizing your thinking about spiritual interventions and helping you remember the wide range of intervention options you might use. Particularly if your work with a client has gotten stuck, you can use this rubric to look for a way of helping your client that might have slipped off your radar.

All spiritual interventions are four-dimensional. Whenever we say or do something to try to help a client—whenever we make an intervention—we are working on one side or the other of these four axes:

- Leveraging an internal resource, or leveraging an external resource
- Leveraging an implicitly spiritual resource, or leveraging an explicitly spiritual one
- Inviting the client to try something in session, right here with us, or inviting the client to try something out of session, after they leave
- Aiming our intervention at the left hemisphere of the client's brain, or aiming it at the right hemisphere

(This is not a book about brain science, but let me say a few words about this last bullet point. The human brain, as you know, has two sides, the left and right, connected by a broad band of nerves called the corpus callosum. For many years, neuroscience taught that the left side of our brain is the home of language, logic, and linear thinking—all words that begin with the letter L, conveniently—and the right is home to intuitive, imagistic thinking. The left brain, the science held, notices details and puts things in categories—this or that—while the right brain notices things as a whole, in relationship and connectedness. In recent years, neuroscience has revised this picture somewhat, having learned that both sides of the brain are working at all times, whether we're solving a math problem or writing a song.

This revision noted, the idea that there are two ways of thinking, two ways of orienting to reality, still expresses a human truth. Even though, biologically speaking, these two ways of thinking don't neatly divide across the two hemispheres, it is still therapeutically useful to distinguish between them. I think of it this way: the left brain is where we know what we

already know, so interventions aimed at the left hemisphere ask clients to do something they already do or
tell us something they already know. The right brain is
where we know in the present moment, and interventions aimed there are more experimental and experiential in nature, inviting our clients to soften the edges
of habit and allow a new-in-this-moment experience to
occur.)

Here is a shorthand version of the four dimensions:

Internal resource	← →	External resource
Implicit resource	← →	Explicit resource
In-session	← →	Out-of-session
Left-brain	← →	Right-brain

And here are some examples to illustrate:

If a client becomes emotionally dysregulated in your office,
and you offer him a mindfulness practice to help him regulate—notice your feet, notice your legs, notice your breath—
the intervention you have used is

- Internal, because you've directed his attention inwardly
- Implicit, because calling attention to feet, legs, and
  breath does not employ overt religious language
- In-session, because he's trying it here in the office
  with you
- Right-brain, because he's paying attention to experience without trying to categorize it or verbalize about it

Now imagine the same client, but instead of offering a
mindfulness practice, you offer to say aloud some words of
Scripture he has previously told you are important to him: "Be

still and know I am God." You ask him to notice what happens inside as you repeat the words several times. The intervention you are using here is

- Internal, because you're directing his attention inwardly
- Explicit, because you're repeating words of Scripture;
- In-session, because you're doing it right now
- Right-brain, because, once again, he's paying attention to experience without trying to categorize it or verbalize about it

Now imagine a different client talking with you about how lonely she is. You know she's a churchgoer, and you ask her to make a list of people from her church with whom she might want to do something in the next two weeks. The intervention you're using here is

- External, because the resource involved is outside herself: people from her church
- Explicit, because the resource is connected to an explicit spiritual community
- Out-of-session, because she'll be taking action after she leaves the office
- Left-brain, because making a list is paying attention to something already known

One more. Imagine a client trying to make a decision about whether to change jobs. She feels anxious and confused about what to do. You've done some spiritual assessment, and she's told you she feels spiritually at her best when she's working in her garden and cooking slow, elaborate meals. If you reminded her of that, and then wondered aloud if it might help her to do as much of those activities as she possibly can over the next two weeks, the intervention you'd be using is

- External, because gardening and cooking are actions she takes to connect her to things external to herself: dirt, sunlight, pots and pans
- Implicit, because gardening and cooking are not explicitly spiritual
- Out-of-session, since she'll do these things after she leaves
- Left-brain, since she's making a mental note to do this later

On the other hand, if you reminded her that she's told you she feels spiritually at her best when she's gardening and cooking, and then asked her to imagine being in her garden right now—smelling the soil, feeling the sun on her back, hearing the hoe scratching around in the dirt—and notice what starts to happen in her body as she imagines that, this intervention would be

- Internal, since she's doing all this in her mind, rather than actually being in the garden
- Implicit, since gardening is implicitly spiritual
- In-session, since you're asking her to notice her body here and now, with you
- Right-brain, because she's noticing without trying to categorize or verbalize

All interventions are experiments. We try them, notice what happens, and adjust from there. When we have done a good-enough assessment, we usually know which approach, in each dimension, will best serve our client. But if our intervention misses the mark or falls flat, sometimes all that's needed is adjustment in one of these four dimensions.

Many therapists find this four-dimensions rubric helpful in self-supervision. If we are working effectively with a diverse group of clients, we will likely be using interventions from both ends of all four axes. Sometimes, though, we may be uncomfortable with a particular approach: using the client's explicit spiritual language, for example, or working in a more experiential, right-brain-focused way. Think about the spiritual interventions you use most often in your practice and describe them using the four dimensions. Are any sides of any of the four dimensions underrepresented? What do you make of that? With whom can you talk to about it?

CONCLUSION

In this chapter, I've described some interventions you might use to leverage spiritual resources that seem to be positive, helpful, and adaptive in your clients' lives. There are many, many others, not to mention infinite variations on the ones I've included, but what I've described here will get you started.

Remember that *a good intervention is an informed experiment*—informed by assessment, offered with some reasonable expectation that it is a good fit for this client at this moment, yet always an experiment, the impact of which will not be known until we try it. So as you intervene, watch what happens, keep assessing, and adjust from there.

8

....

Working with
Spiritual Struggles

Spiritual Interventions, Part 2

IN THE LAST CHAPTER WE TALKED ABOUT HOW TO AMPLIFY
healthy spiritual resources to help clients stabilize and heal.
But spirituality is not always and only a source of support and
strength. Sometimes it is a source of struggle.

Imagine growing up in a religious tradition, going to a
small college affiliated with that tradition, marrying someone,
going to church, raising your children, and spending most of
your social time all within that tight religious world. Once in
a while you'd feel the foundation crack just a bit—little doubts
here and there—but you were always able to caulk them over
quickly before they opened any wider and caused you much
trouble. Then a loved one got horribly sick and didn't recover,
or a spiritual mentor crashed and burned, or an outside-the-
tribe friendship at work grew to the point that you could no
longer stomach thinking that this person you really like is

going to hell because she doesn't believe what you believe. And one morning you wake up and realize you don't believe it anymore. You wish you could, but you can't. It's a sham. And just like that, your entire world—the things you believe, the ways you spend your time, your closest friends, everything—is lost to you. You're terrified, isolated, angry, and sad.

Or imagine not growing up in a religious tradition. You knew people who were religious or spiritual, but none of that ever made sense to you. You were a "this world" person, you worked sixty hours a week and loved it, you got things done. And then you retired. Now there are no big problems to solve, no ladders to climb, no company intrigue to occupy your imagination. The meaning system that organized your world and oriented you in it—manage, strive, succeed—is gone, and you have no idea what to do with yourself, no idea what makes a day a good day, no idea what the value of your life is. You wake every morning, eat your cereal, flip the channels, and wonder what the heck you're going to do for the next twenty years.

Or imagine your faith teaches you it's not OK to be gay, but it's clear to you that you are. Or it's not OK to divorce, but your marriage is killing you.

All people experience spiritual struggles. Some are explicitly spiritual, others are implicitly spiritual, but sooner or later, everyone encounters the kind of loss, transition, vulnerability, and chaos that rocks the foundation of our world and hurls us into the whirlwind of "Why?" and "What now?"

Struggles like these cause great distress and anguish for our clients—and clients being tossed about in the storm of struggle can cause great distress and anguish for therapists. Colleagues often tell me how uneasy they feel being the person their clients talk with about spiritual struggles, particularly explicit spiritual struggles. "They're asking questions I can't answer," therapists tell me. "I'm not a spiritual expert, and I don't know what to say. It's stressful to be the one they're looking to for help."

And I say back, to them and to you: yes, absolutely. It's a very difficult spot to be in. People come to us with questions we can't possibly answer. Life has just blown their world to bits. They're hurting, scared, and uncertain, miles beyond the borders of the world they've known and trusted until now. They feel disoriented, panicky, and hopeless, and we want to offer something that helps their head stop spinning and their heart stop hurting. But what can we offer? What is there to say, with certainty, about matters of mystery?

What's important, of course, is not having answers. Most of the time there just aren't any of those anyway. What's important is accompanying strugglers into the unknown, staying with them while their world is reeling, validating and normalizing their experience, resisting whatever temptation we might feel to offer some easy but false answer, asking good questions, being a calm voice that lets them know they're not alone, and staying with them while they learn to integrate this struggle into a larger way of being in the world. If this chapter has a central message, it is this: *accompaniment instead of answers.*

It takes courage and humility to do this—to offer accompaniment instead of answers—and the rest of this chapter is about supporting you in being courageous and humble. I'll talk with you about why it's important for therapists to be available to help our clients with spiritual struggles, give an overview of different kinds of spiritual struggles, offer some principles to guide your work, and share two clinical illustrations: one of an explicit spiritual struggle, one of an implicit spiritual struggle.

WHY SPIRITUAL STRUGGLES MATTER FOR THERAPISTS

In the field of psychology, the person who has contributed most to my understanding of spiritual struggles is Ken Pargament.

He writes about spiritual struggles in *Spiritually Integrated Psychotherapy* and is currently completing, with Julie Exline, an entire book about spiritual struggles. After you read this chapter and are ready to go deeper into the topic, Pargament should be the very next source you consult. Here, briefly, are some of his primary ideas.

Pargament defines *spiritual struggles* as "experiences of tension, strain, and conflict about sacred matters within oneself, with others, and with the divine,"[1] and he cites research—his own and that of others—showing that spiritual struggles are fairly common. Spiritual struggles have been found among people from a variety of religious traditions, including Muslims,[2] Christians,[3] and Jews.[4] In a study of patients with advanced cancer, for instance, 58 percent said they were experiencing a spiritual struggle.[5]

Pargament explains that psychological problems can cause spiritual struggles—a person's depression, for example, can make her feel that God has abandoned her—and that spiritual struggles can cause psychological problems—a person's spiritual despair can make her feel depressed.

Perhaps most importantly, Pargament asserts that while some people end up healthier and experience a greater sense of wellbeing as a result of their spiritual struggles—their struggles become an occasion for growth—sometimes the opposite happens.[6] And one of the key predictors of whether spiritual struggles become occasions for growth or decline is the kind of support persons receive in the midst of their struggles.

That's where you come in. Even though you might not see yourself as a spiritual expert, you may be the only person your clients feel safe speaking to about their spiritual struggles. They may face rejection, shaming, coercion, or ostracism if they voice these issues in their religious community. So uneasy or not, you might be the person they choose to talk with, and that's why this chapter is so important.

KINDS OF SPIRITUAL STRUGGLES

Here is a partial list of the kinds of spiritual struggles people often want to talk about in psychotherapy:

- Guilt and forgiveness
- Resentment and forgiveness
- Feeling unworthy or undeserving
- Losing faith, or feeling doubt about beliefs
- Losing a spiritual community
- Losing confidence in a spiritual leader or mentor
- Feeling let down by, disappointed in, angry at, or cut off from God
- Feeling attacked by the devil or some other evil force
- A disturbing spiritual experience (like the one described in the last chapter: Jasmine encountering the spirit of her deceased father)
- Difficulties with a spiritual practice, for example, racing thoughts during meditation
- Wrestling with a moral choice or a spiritual "vice"
- Questions about meaning and purpose
- Making sense of suffering

Any of these struggles can be occasioned by loss, illness, trauma, or overwhelming stress—things that happen to us, apart from any choice on our part—but we should also remember that spiritual struggles are sometimes freely chosen. All spiritual traditions teach that the spiritual life is a journey, that to become our truest selves, we must live beyond many of the habits, attachments, and securities of our less-than-truest selves. Journeys like these can be frightening, painful, and costly. Even so, many adherents of all spiritual traditions choose them willingly.

Pargament sorts these assorted struggles into three categories:

- **Interpersonal struggles.** These are "spiritual conflicts and tensions with families, friends, and congregations," including "gossiping, cliquishness, hypocrisy on the part of clergy and members, and disagreements with church doctrine."[7]
- **Intrapersonal struggles.** These include inner struggles with meaning, doubt, uncertainty, sense of worth, and sense of purpose. They also include struggles with moral issues and feelings of guilt and shame.[8]
- **Supernatural struggles.** These include feeling punished by God, abandoned by God, or angry with God, as well as feeling tormented or tempted by some malevolent spiritual force, like the devil.[9]

But you will recognize—and Pargament does too—that most struggles do not fit neatly into any one category.

SOME PRINCIPLES TO WORK BY

I've already said that our job is not to provide answers. Our job is to be a supportive accompanying presence for our clients as they grow into their own answers, to stick with them as they make their way to some resolution, to be a human being who stays alongside and does not leave them alone. And I've said that this requires courage and humility on our part.

But accompaniment without answers does not mean accompaniment without wisdom. There are some principles and strategies we work by that are of great benefit to spiritual strugglers. It's likely you already have your own supply of these, but in this section I want to name a few of mine.

Connect with the Struggler

Sometimes a spiritual struggle is so compelling and interesting to us—Why do bad things happen to good people? How can I atone for my mistakes? How can I pray when I don't believe in anything?—that we get captivated by the content of the struggle and forget about the person who's experiencing it. Don't let this happen to you!

Spiritual struggles often have a cognitive component, involving and affecting what people believe and how they think about life. Even so, spiritual struggles are emotional, limbic experiences more than they are cognitive, cortical experiences. People with spiritual struggles feel confused, afraid, and alone. They are grieving, ashamed, or angry. And while there are often points where we join a client in conversation about belief and meaning, these more cognitive conversations are of little impact if we have not made connection with the client's emotional experience.

So a good rule of thumb is: *connect with the struggler first, not the struggle.* Let there be a free flow of empathy, respect, curiosity, and care between you and your client. Make sure your struggler feels met as a person, not as a problem to be solved.

Normalize, Normalize, Normalize

One of the worst parts of spiritual struggle is feeling that the reason you're going through it is because there's something wrong with you. If only you were a better person, if only you had more faith, if only you had done this or that differently, maybe none of this would be happening. Therefore, one of the most important things we offer clients is reassurance that what they're experiencing is a normal part of the human experience and a normal part of spiritual experience. They're not wrong to be feeling what they're feeling or thinking what they're thinking.

We normalize the struggler's experience most easily by offering ordinary, uncomplicated words of assurance: "That makes sense." "Yes. Of course." "That's so real." "That's so human."

We normalize by simply not flinching or pulling away from our clients. Our embodied, caring presence conveys that the struggle they are experiencing is one that can be lived with and engaged.

We also normalize by linking our clients' experience with the experience of some spiritual authority they might respect. In the past week alone, when writing this chapter, I have called upon the words of Jesus, Mother Teresa, and Bruce Springsteen. From Jesus: "My God, my God, why have you forsaken me?"[10] From Mother Teresa: "I am told God loves me, and yet the reality of the darkness and coldness and emptiness is so great that nothing touches my soul."[11] And from the Boss, speaking about the death of his friend and bandmate Clarence Clemmons: "[It] created a hole in me that's never going to be filled. And that's life, once you get to a certain age. You're going to end up with a life that has a lot of holes in it."[12]

Stay with It

Staying with struggle is not easy. Our clients will sometimes want to avoid the pain of their struggle or distract themselves from it as quickly as possible; and we will sometimes want to do the same. But the way through struggle is indeed usually *through* it, not around it, and one of the most important things we do is help clients stay with their struggle a little longer—to not run from it quite so fast—so that some degree of resolution, integration, or expansion can happen. Often, it is the sound of our voice or the look in our eye that helps people believe their struggle is survivable, our refusal to mouth some platitude that allows clients to seek deeper and more functional beliefs, and the difficult questions we are brave enough to ask that give our clients courage to keep noticing and speaking the truth of their experience. Your willingness to walk with clients in the valley of the shadow of struggle, to match their pace and not rush them, even sometimes to slow them down, is a gift that can change their lives—and maybe yours as well.

Follow the Energy

Spiritual struggles are a bit like labor pains: they're agonizing, yet sometimes they're necessary for something new to be born. That makes you a bit of a midwife, supporting your client while she labors.

Remember that the contractions of labor come and go. They amp up in intensity, then they subside. Much as midwives follow the energy of the mother in labor, we must follow the energy of our clients engaged in spiritual struggle. Sometimes "follow the energy" means going deep with clients—helping them "stay with it" as long as it takes. Other times it means taking a break, giving you and your client a chance to catch your breath, affirm the good labor that's happening, and prepare yourselves to ride the next wave.

Engage All the Building Blocks

In the last chapter I named five building blocks of experience—"thoughts (cognitions), emotions, perceptions (internally generated images, tastes, smells, touch, and sounds), body movements, and body sensations"[13]—and illustrated how we can increase the impact of a spiritual resource by helping clients notice that resource in as many ways as possible. The same principle applies to working with spiritual struggles: engage as many of the building blocks as possible.

People in the midst of spiritual struggle get stuck most often in the realms of cognition and emotion. They're trying to comprehend the incomprehensible and think their way through the unthinkable. Or they're overwhelmed by feelings like sadness, anger, and guilt. When we recognize our clients are floundering in either of these ways—stuck in their heads or overwhelmed by emotion—a good way to help is to shift attention to one of the other building blocks. Thus, if a client is going round in circles grappling with the cognitive dimension of a struggle, try shifting his attention to emotion, or to sensation in his body. If a client seems stuck in emotion—hopeless, angry, guilty, or such—try shifting her attention to cognition or to some impulse to move. "If that guilty feeling could speak," for instance, "what would it say?" (a shift to cognition). Or "If that guilty feeling could express itself through your body in any way, if it could move your body, what would it do?" (a shift to body sensation or body movement). These shifts in attention often help clients get moving again.

Check Your Four Dimensions

Also in the last chapter, I introduced a concept called "interventions in four dimensions." I said that all interventions involve one side or the other of four axes:

Internal resource	← →	External resource
Implicit resource	← →	Explicit resource
In-session	← →	Out-of-session
Left-brain	← →	Right-brain

I suggested that when we get stuck with a client, it's helpful to notice whether we're working too one-sidedly in any of these dimensions. This way of thinking about your work is also helpful when addressing spiritual struggles. Is your client trying to resolve a spiritual struggle using a mostly right-brain approach? Let's see what happens if you invite her left brain to engage the process a little. Is your client trying to work his way through a spiritual struggle by getting other people to tell him what to think and do—leaning mainly on external resources, including you? Try inviting him to remember and explore some of his internal resources.

Remember That You're Not Alone

Last but not least, remember that there is time-tested spiritual genius available to help you.

All the great religions were born of struggle: Hinduism from a clash of cultures, when the Indo-Aryan people migrated into the Indus Valley; Buddhism from Gautama's disturbance at the realities of death and suffering; Judaism from the experience of slavery and oppression in Egypt; Christianity from the execution of Jesus and the persecution of his followers; and Islam from the revelations given to an orphan, Muhammad, whose receipt of the revelations that became the Quran included a three-year period of depression and intense spiritual struggle. And all these great religions offer wisdom about facing spiritual struggle with honesty and authenticity.[14]

Your client may be part of one or more of these religious traditions, and part of your supporting them in their struggle is helping them draw upon the resources of their tradition. You don't have to be an expert in their tradition, but your respect for that tradition and your curiosity about it can help you frame questions like these:

- Are there perspectives in your religion about this struggle?
- Are there stories, religious figures, passages of Scripture, music, or other things that bring any light to this?
- Are there people you know, inside or outside your religion, who've already asked these questions?
- What does God understand about your situation and what you're feeling that nobody else does?[15]

You may be part of a religious tradition too, and you can draw upon its wisdom to guide your work with your client. You won't impose the wisdom of your tradition, but you can use it to help you do your work. I'll be saying more about this in part 3 of this book, but I'll offer a short word here about what I mean. In Christianity, there is the teaching that we find our lives by losing our lives, that the way to resurrection is through dying. I rarely name this teaching explicitly to my clients, and when I do it is always after learning, through spiritual assessment, that my client is a Christian. But this teaching about the nature of reality helps me stay connected with clients who are in the anguish of struggle.

Even if you're not connected to a religious tradition, fear not. You're still a human being, and all these traditions belong to the human family. The light they cast is still available to you, and the stories, metaphors, practices, and saints of all these traditions can support you as you support your clients. And representatives of those traditions—clergy, chaplains, spiritual directors, and others—are only a phone call away.

CLINICAL ILLUSTRATIONS

In the remainder of this chapter, I want to let you see these principles in action. I'll offer one illustration with someone who thinks of her spiritual struggle in explicitly spiritual terms and a second with someone who does not. In both, I hope you'll recognize that I'm not providing answers. I'm working with what's presented, following the energy and wisdom of the client, and occasionally giving things an experimental nudge.

Struggling with Divorce

This first example is of a woman whose spiritual struggle concerns her marriage and her relationship with God. This is one of the more common spiritual struggles people bring to therapy: "My marriage is horrible and I want to leave. My religion says I shouldn't. What should I do?" You have probably worked with this issue any number of times in your practice, or you may have wrestled with it in your own life. If so, you know that many religious people believe that marriage is sacred: a promise they've made not just to their partner but to God and to their faith community. So in addition to the emotional, social, financial, and logistical turmoil that is part of most every divorce, in addition to the devastating feelings of failure and shame that people sometimes feel, there can also be a sense of disappointing or perhaps even angering God, and becoming a second-class person in—even a total outcast from—one's spiritual community.

You may have your own spiritually informed values and perspectives about divorce. Perhaps you believe people take their marriage vows too lightly, and religion is right to hold people accountable to their promises. Or maybe you know how easy it is to make a mistake in choosing a mate, and you think religion should support people in moving past their mistakes and into a better life. But whatever your personal opinions are, you recognize that effective and ethical practice means supporting your clients in doing their own work and finding their own decision, not trying to persuade them to see things your way or do what you would want.

Marie was recently separated from her husband of twelve years. They had two children and had been seeing a counselor together at their church. She felt the need for some individual counseling, and a friend from work gave her my name.

On the intake form, she wrote that she was coming for counseling because she was depressed. But when I asked her in session what she wanted help with, she said, "What I should feel and what I do feel are not the same." I asked her to say more, and she said, "I *should* want to be married, I *should* love my husband, I *should* want to keep things stable for my kids, but I *don't* love my husband and I *don't* want to stay married." Then she added, "If this is what God wants me to want, to stay married, why don't I want it?"

It turns out Marie did meet criteria for moderate depression, and she was already taking an SSRI antidepressant. But the main thing she wanted to focus on in therapy was her spiritual struggle. She had become confused about God—what God is like and what God expected of her—and she wanted to sort through how her beliefs about God and her relationship with God should affect this decision about her marriage.

I asked her to tell me more about herself, her marriage, and her faith. Marie described herself as an evangelical Christian. She had attended church regularly throughout her adulthood. Her marriage, she said, had been difficult for a long time. She's not a naturally warm person, she said, and her husband had wanted more connection with her for as long as they'd been married. She thinks she's been a frustrating person for him to be married to, and he has been critical about how nonexpressive she is. A few years ago he said he wanted to end the marriage. That's not what Marie wanted, but she agreed to a separation anyway. As soon as she agreed, he changed his mind, and they stayed together. But he continued to be hard on her, to be critical of "who she's not," and to express frustration that she wouldn't or couldn't change for him. He was sometimes openly critical but more often critical in passive-aggressive ways, and it had finally worn her down.

Then one day, about a year before her first appointment with me, Marie was sitting in church, thinking about leaving and praying about what to do. She told God she wanted to leave but that she was worried about how a divorce would affect the children. Then she felt God say, "I can take care of them. You have to let him go." That afternoon she told her husband she wanted to leave, but he begged her not to do that. He asked her to go to counseling with him, and she agreed.

The counselor they saw told Marie that it was not OK for her to leave, since there was no biblically justifiable cause to end the marriage.[16] Marie accepted the counselor's advice and stayed for another seven months. She and her husband kept seeing the counselor, and Marie grew sadder and wearier. Eventually she told her husband and her counselor, "I just need a brief separation. Not a divorce, just a little time to myself."

Her husband agreed to this and moved in with his parents, who lived nearby. It was at this point that she came to her first appointment with me.

In our second session together, Marie described her struggle this way. There's a side of her, she said, that wants to please God and believes that pleasing God means staying in her marriage. That side of her worries that she won't be able do so, and she was tearful as she told me about it. Then she talked about another side of herself. She described it as a barrier that she could actually feel, on the right side of her body. She said it was like a piece of Saran Wrap, and whenever she tried moving toward her husband, even in her mind, she could not get past this barrier. The barrier would not let her go in the direction she thought she needed to go to please God, which confused and frustrated her.

I asked if she felt curious about the barrier and if she'd be willing to explore it. She said she was, so I invited her to ask the barrier if it had a job and, if it did, what that job was.[17]

Marie:	It's there to protect me.
Russell:	Protect you from what?
Marie:	From a mistake. If it's not there and I go back to my husband, my heart will be destroyed. [Her eyes well up with tears.]
Russell:	And what are your tears saying?
Marie:	I'm just feeling so grateful to this barrier, that it wants to protect my heart.
Russell:	Yes. So maybe just let it know that. That you feel grateful toward it.
Marie:	[Silence] Now it's saying, "Don't let guilt hurt me."
Russell:	"Don't let guilt hurt me."
Marie:	Right. There's this strong feeling of guilt about leaving him.

Russell: And can you feel that physically, too, like the Saran Wrap?

Marie: Yes. It's a heaviness in my heart. Like a weight.

Russell: OK. So maybe focus on that for a minute, very gently, that weight, that guilt, and ask it if it has a job too.

Marie: It does. Its job is to keep me from being a bad person.

Russell: And ask it how it does that job. What does it do to keep you from being a bad person?

Marie: [Silence] It tells me things I shouldn't do. It says if I do them then I'm a bad person. And it gets very heavy in me, like a giant immovable boulder.

Russell: And how does that affect you, the way guilt does this job?

Marie: It's really pretty horrible.

Russell: Right. I can feel that. It really wants to help you, to help you be a good person, but the way it does that is really heavy on you.

Marie: Yes.

Russell: So maybe, if this feels authentic to you, maybe thank it for wanting to help you be a good person, and also let it know how heavy it feels in you, and how hard it feels to the Saran Wrap part of you that wants to keep your heart from being destroyed but that feels like guilt could hurt it.

Marie: [Silence, a softening of her face]

Russell: What's happening now?

Marie: I can feel the guilt lightening up in my heart. It still wants to help me do right, but it feels easier in me somehow.

We are working here with an explicitly spiritual struggle, but since spirituality is connected to and inseparable from all the other dimensions of our existence—thoughts, feelings, physicality, relationships—we are doing spiritual work whenever we work with any of these other dimensions. I point this out to those of you who worry that you're not spiritual enough to work with spiritual struggles and to those of you who might really enjoy having an explicit spiritual conversation with your clients. Even when your client's struggle is an explicitly spiritual one, as it was with Marie, you don't have to have something spiritually amazing to say. Sometimes, in fact, getting into the cognitive dimensions of the struggle too quickly or too deeply only reinforces the stuckness. Just pay attention, stay curious, and keep engaging.

In her third session, Marie told me that, over the weekend, her husband asked her to let him move back in. "How can we work on our marriage," he said, "if we're not spending any time together?" She told him, very clearly and very easily, "I can't right now." He then resumed the passive-aggressive cold-shoulder approach that was his pattern, and she thought, *He hasn't changed.*

Also in this third session, she said to me, for the first time, "I want a divorce." I am always on the lookout for statements of clarity like this—"I think," "I feel," "I want," "I won't"—and I usually mirror them back to clients and invite them to test the truth and wisdom of these declarations. So I asked Marie to check inside and notice what she felt and heard when she said those words to herself: "I want a divorce." She said she felt a warmth in her chest.

Russell:	So maybe just stay with that warmth. Let it happen. And notice what happens next.
Marie:	I feel God telling me, "It's OK. It's OK to get this divorce."

Russell: And when you feel that warmth, and when you feel God speaking to you this way, what happens then?

Marie: I feel very grateful. [Silence] Emotional. [Silence] Relaxed. [She opens her eyes and looks at me.]

Russell: "Grateful. Emotional. Relaxed."

Marie: This is the first time I've felt God in twelve months. Since that time in church when God told me I had to let him go, that God would take care of the kids, but then I stayed. After that I stopped being able to hear from God. And this is the first time I've heard from God since then.

Russell: Wow. So just let that soak in. Take your time. [Silence] Mind if I check with you about one other thing?

Marie: No. Go ahead.

Russell: The way you're feeling now, connected with God, warm in your body, hearing that it's OK to get this divorce, I wonder what happens if you imagine your husband asking you to reconsider, or someone telling you that it's not OK with God for you to get a divorce.

Marie: It's OK. I still feel clear. There's no clinching up about that.

Russell: And what about the guilt part, that you connected with last week, that wants you to be a good person. How's it doing?

Marie: It knows I'm a good person.

Marie came six more times over the next four months. During these months she and her husband worked out a separation agreement. She stopped therapy before her divorce was finalized, but she returned two years later for a few sessions when she began wanting to date again.

GRIEF, GUILT, ANGER, AND MEANING

Now I want to illustrate working with a spiritual struggle with a client who does not consider himself spiritual or religious. One of the things I'm saying again and again in this book is that spiritual issues are not always explicitly spiritual. It takes eyes to see and ears to hear, but spiritual issues are embedded in everyday life—and in spiritually integrated psychotherapy, it is important to treat the sacred as sacred however it appears, even if it is not explicitly spiritual.

The client in the following example has experienced a traumatic loss—his son's death by suicide—and his struggles are those people often feel in the wake of such a tragedy: grief, guilt, and difficulty finding meaning. This man is a current client. His anguish is nowhere near resolved, and this is one of the reasons I have chosen to include his story: working with spiritual struggles means ending lots and lots of sessions without a sense of resolution, and part of our work is to help hold that unresolved feeling with our clients.

This example also illustrates three other things I think are important: (1) that we can engage a spiritual struggle very deeply without ever using explicit spiritual language; (2) that our clients possess great wisdom for moving through struggle, and a large part of our work is to watch for this wisdom to arise and to collaborate with it; and (3) that while following the client's wisdom and energy is helpful, it can also be helpful, sometimes, to give a little nudge.

Jim is seventy-two, married to Linda, and four years into retirement after a career as a home-builder. He does not see himself as religious or spiritual.

Jim's only child, James, died by suicide three years ago. James had struggled for years with depression and addiction. Jim loved his son dearly and had spent much time and energy the past twenty years trying to help him. James' death is a great blow, and Jim's ongoing grief, lethargy, and guilt are the reasons he has come for therapy. He said he felt stuck and decided he should try getting some help.

Jim is ambivalent about coming to therapy. He does not like feeling his feelings, and he wonders if therapy can really help. Nevertheless, the therapeutic alliance seems strong. As of this writing, we have been meeting every other week for five months. He seems to like me—he teases me in a good-natured way—and he talks openly about his sadness, guilt, and purposelessness. He is psychologically insightful and has observed a gap between his head and heart. He knows in his head, for instance, that he could have done nothing more to help his son, but in his heart, he continues to hold himself responsible.

Jim says he feels immense sadness, cries about once a week, and feels a strong sense of guilt—not just for being unable to save his son from terminal depression but also for having hidden the severity of his son's depression from his wife, Linda. She knew a bit, but Jim had most of the contact with James, and he did not let his wife know how bad things had become. At the time, this felt like a kind thing to do for her—and for James, who did not react well to his mother's worry. But given that their son had died, Jim feels like he denied his wife the opportunity to know him fully and to help if she could have.

In addition to missing his son, Jim also misses the "reason for living" that his son provided. After Jim retired, caring for his son was one of the few things he found meaningful. He walks every day, plays golf with friends once a week, and volunteers one day a week at a local food bank, but he does not feel inspired by any of it. He is not suicidal, but he does not know what he's living for anymore.

Jim does not believe in God and would not say he is angry with God or wrestling with God. But he is angry and wrestling all the same—with Universal Justice and Fairness, with Reality, with Life—with whatever he might call all that's bigger than he is and that he can't control. He feels like a man holding a grudge. He is saying no to his own living, which I regard as the implicit spiritual dimension of Jim's struggle.

There is no loss like losing a child, and no loss like losing a loved one to suicide. I have not lost a child, but I have lost a family member to suicide, so I feel a strong connection to this part of Jim's struggle. At times it is hard for me to "stay with it" with Jim, but accompanying him in his grief is also an experience of healing for me.

The following exchange happened in the last fifteen minutes of our tenth session.

Jim: I don't believe in God, but if I did, I'd be angry at him.

Russell: Yes. [Nodding]

Jim: I guess I'm mad at life. [One of the principles of working with spiritual struggles, as with other issues in psychotherapy, is to follow the client's energy. The energy here is anger, and so I want to respond to the anger and, if possible, help him connect with it across as many building blocks as possible.]

Russell: How about just feel the mad? [Silence] Sometimes it's hard and frustrating not to know where to direct the mad. So feel that too.

Jim: I don't see the point in that. [There is a bit of aggression in his words here. I have felt previously with Jim that he likes a bit of aggressive back-and-forth. Perhaps he is accustomed to this from his work as a builder. Sometimes it is playful, but here it feels *more serious. I meet his pushback with a pushback of my own.]*

Russell: The point is: your anger is gonna help make a way forward for you.

Jim: I'm not sure I want a way forward.

Russell: Yes, I feel that in you, and it makes sense.

Jim: What do you mean?

Russell: I mean, I feel that there's a part of you that doesn't want to move forward. But another part of you does. I mean, you're sitting in a frickin therapist's office. That's why you came. But there's a disagreement in you. Between the part of you that wants a chance to live the rest of your life and the part of you that says you don't have a right to that.

Jim: Aaaaaaaa. [Shaking his head, frustrated and annoyed] Dammit dammit dammit. *[Jim was not yelling, but there was a lot of irritation in his voice. Irritation, of course, is energy, and "follow the energy" here means following the irritation, even amplifying it.]*

Russell: Dammit what?

Jim: Dammit, I don't know. [Still irritated]

Russell: Well, then, don't know. But keep dammiting.

Jim: Dammit.

Russell: Yes. Dammit dammit!

Jim: Dammit!

Russell: This is real. You're feeling something you can't put into words. Dammit's the best you've got right now. I get it. But stay with it if you can. *[One of the tried-and-true-but-underused resources for grief and struggle in the Judeo-Christian tradition*

*is the practice of lament. The wisdom of those com-
munities is, "When heartache happens, speak and
sing your hurt into the heart of your community."
Around 40 percent of the Bible's psalms are psalms
of lament: "How long, O Lord? Will you hide your
face from me forever?"[18] And there are laments in
other parts of the Bible too: "Why did I not perish at
birth, and die as I came from the womb?"[19] Jim does
not have a community with which to do this, but at
this point in the session, he and I had fallen into an
implicitly spiritual litany of lament.]*

Jim:	Dammit. [His energy is deflating.]
Russell:	Dammit what?

Jim:	Dammit, I miss my son.
Russell:	Yes.

Jim:	Dammit, I wish he hadn't done that.
Russell:	Yes.

Jim:	Dammit, I hate the way this works. *[I don't know what he means here, but he is in a flow, and I don't want to interrupt it by asking him to explain.]*
Russell:	Yes.

Jim:	It's wrong, dammit. He tried. And I tried.
Russell:	Yes.

Jim:	And it didn't matter. *[I actually am bothered by his words here: "It didn't matter." And again I don't know what he means. But it feels like there is momentum in his processing, and I don't want to get in its way by asking him to explain. I return to these words in our next session, as I describe below, but for now I just keep him moving.]*
Russell:	Yes.

Jim: I just want to punch something.
Russell: Yes. Feel it.

Jim: Aaaaaa. [With irritation]
Russell: Yes.

Jim: Aaaaaaaaaaaa. [With greater irritation]
Russell: Yes.

Jim: [Silence] I'm an old man.
Russell: You are.

Jim: My knees are shot.
Russell: Yes.

Jim: And I couldn't stop my son from dying.
Russell: No, you could not.

Jim: [Silence] Dammit.
Russell: Dammit.

We were at the end of our time, and we sat together in silence for a few minutes before I told him we needed to stop.

When Jim returned two weeks later, we exchanged a bit of small talk as we settled into our seats. Then I asked him what had happened after he left.

Jim: Oh God. I was so exhausted. I hated you for putting me through that. [He says this in a friendly way.]
Russell: You're welcome.

Jim: [He laughs.] I was so tired. I just went home and took a nap.
Russell: Yeah, that was intense. But what was the next day like? And the days after that?

Jim: Um. You know. Just normal days. I went for walks. I ate dinner with Linda. I went to the food bank. I possibly felt a little more energy.

Russell: OK. More energy, like how?

Jim: I finally put my garden to bed.
Russell: Oh. I didn't know you have a garden.

Then Jim talked with me about his garden. I don't want to make overly much of this metaphor, and I did not say any of this to him, but it was not lost on me that in the week following the experience of lament, Jim had engaged in at least one activity that we might call "cooperating with life." He had returned to his relationship with the earth, with the seasons, and with things that grow.

A bit later in this session, I returned to a comment Jim had made the previous week. Here I am not particularly following his lead or his energy. I am introducing a theme he and I have discussed before—the meaning of his life now that he is retired and his son has died—but that was not in play at this point in the session.

Russell: I want to ask you about something you said last week.

Jim: As long as we don't have to get all intense.

Russell: Well, I don't know that that's entirely up to me. [Playfully] But actually, that makes me want to ask you a different question. Do you regret what happened in here last week?

Jim: No. Not really. It was just hard.

Russell: Yes. It really was. And that makes me want to ask you what you'd say happened in here last week, in you, for you?

Jim: Aaaa. I don't know. I guess I just let myself feel mad at something other than myself. I'm not sure what that something is. But something besides just me.

Russell: Yeah. That makes sense. That's how it felt to me too. [Silence]

Jim: So is that what you wanted to ask me about?

Russell: Oh. Right. No. Thanks for reminding me. I wanted to ask you about when you said, "It didn't matter." You said James had tried, and you had tried, but it didn't matter. Do you remember that?

Jim: Yeah. Sorta.

Russell: So those words really struck me. A lot of what happened in that session struck me. But I wanted to ask you about those words. "He tried. I tried. And it didn't matter." What did you mean by that?

Jim: I mean that it didn't help. It didn't change the outcome. It didn't stop him from killing himself.

Russell: OK. That's what I thought you meant. But can I just ask? James still killed himself. He still died of depression. And you and Linda are living with this giant hole in your lives. But his trying, and your trying, did the trying really not matter?

Jim: I hear you.

Russell: OK. Well—

Jim: I'm an outcomes person. I was a builder, remember?

Russell: Right. [Silence] But were there any other outcomes that came from you and him trying that mattered?

Jim: [Silence] He knew that I loved him.

Russell: That mattered.

Jim: Yes.

Russell: So the thing you showed each other by trying— love . . . that mattered?

Jim: Yes.

Russell: [Silence] Do you still love him?

Jim: He's not here.

Russell: Yes, but when you think of him, do you still love him?

Jim: [Silence] Yes.

Russell: Does that matter?

Jim: I don't know. I'll have to think about that.

Russell: That's fine. [Pause] Just don't think too hard. Mostly just let yourself feel the love and notice how it affects you.

Jim: If you say so.

Russell: That's why you pay me the big bucks. [I smile.]

Jim: Ha! [He smiles.]

Russell: So here's some more. Who else do you love?

Jim: Linda. My brother.

Russell: And does that matter? The love you feel for them?

Jim: Like I said, I'm gonna have to think about that.

Russell: And like I said, don't think too hard. Just notice the effect it has on you and them.

Jim: You're trying to make a point with me, aren't you?

Russell: Yes, I am.

Jim: Well, I'm a businessman. Tell it to me straight.

Russell: Fair enough. [Pause] Give me a minute. [Pause] I've said to you before that it looks like there's a battle going on in you—between the part of you that wants to move forward with your life and the part that says you shouldn't. If James can't, you can't either. I think of that as an honorable battle. The soldiers in it are full of love and grief and guilt and anger and all kinds of other noble feelings.

But to whatever extent you do get to live, choose to live, you're gonna need to have something you think is worth living for. And what I'm hearing from you is that the thing that's worth living for, maybe, one of the things, anyway, is love. The love you feel for Linda and for your brother. The love you live with them. And I'm glad you've got that. Some sense of something that matters. Not everybody does, but I'm glad you do. [Silence] So what I just said, how does it land in you?

Jim: I'll have to think about it. [He and I laugh.] No, seriously, it's something I want to reflect on. There's something there. But I want to reflect on it some more.

Russell: Sounds good. Me too actually. What really matters? To me?

Jim: Well, I'm glad I could help you. [He smiles.]

Russell: Hey. Human beings on a journey. Every one of us.

CONCLUSION

The closing of the conversation above—"Human beings on a journey. Every one of us"—is a good line to help end this chapter on working with spiritual struggles. The essential skill here is the ability to be a human being alongside another human being. We need hearts large enough to hold sorrow and joy, and minds large enough to relax in the presence of ambiguity and paradox. We may at times feel overwhelmed at the intensity of our clients' emotion in the midst of struggle. We may also feel overwhelmed at how unanswerable their questions are. But if we are willing to be human ourselves—to feel, to resonate—and to speak from our humanness, we can make a difference.

Other skills also matter and we have named some of them in this chapter: recognizing implicit spiritual struggles, restraining ourselves from giving answers and trying to fix things quickly, expanding spiritual resources by using all the building blocks and a variety of interventions, and accepting wisdom from your clients', your own, and the world's spiritual traditions.

But the main skill, which is actually a way of being more than a skill, is wholehearted humanness. This also is the main skill in working with harmful religion and spirituality, the topic of the next chapter.

Read on, then, wholehearted human.

9

Working with Harmful Spirituality

Spiritual Interventions, Part 3

I BET YOU WISH WE DIDN'T NEED A CHAPTER ABOUT HARMFUL spirituality and religion. I know I do. I wish there were no such thing as children who were sexually abused by priests, or women who are told to remain in abusive marriages because leaving would be a sin, or suicide bombers who believe that murdering innocent civilians is God's will. I wish there were no such thing as religiously justified prejudice, hatred, or war; or religiously based shame; or spiritual perspectives that diminish joy, pleasure, and healthy risk. I wish there were no people on the planet who think they are bad because they believe God thinks they are bad.

But there are such things, as you well know. Spirituality can be a powerful positive force in the lives of individuals and communities, but it can also be a powerful negative force. Griffith and Griffith say it this way: "An awful irony of human life is the recognition that spiritual beliefs and practices, intended as doorways into the wholeness of life and relationships, can as quickly become doorways to hell."[1]

As therapists, we work with people who are spiritually injured and people who cause spiritual injury. Often these are one and the same. Not all victims of damaging spirituality or religion become perpetrators, but all the perpetrators you'll ever meet were victims first. Usually they have sustained spiritual hurt at some moment in their past, and this is the case in the primary illustration I share later in this chapter. But also, since we can't hurt another person without also hurting ourselves—this is the spiritual truth that underlies what we now call "moral injury"[2]—the injurer is sustaining a self-inflicted spiritual injury in the present.

Working with harmful spirituality and religion is incredibly difficult. It's difficult to witness: it's hard to see harm of any form, but even more when the harm involves something sacred twisted into something malignant. It's difficult to know what to do: it won't just go away if we ignore it, but it usually gets worse if we confront it. And it's difficult to experience the limits of our power as therapists: it's ten times harder to help someone change when their maladaptive thoughts and behavior have the sanction of a religious perspective.

Difficult or not, though, it's part of our job. And in this chapter, I want to help you do this part of your job more effectively. We talked briefly about harmful spirituality and religion in chapter 6, the chapter about spiritual assessment. But here we'll talk more about what harmful spirituality looks like, how it happens, and how to intervene.

A REMINDER ABOUT WHAT WE'RE ASSESSING

One of the things I said in chapter 6 is that, as therapists, we're not in the business of deciding whether our clients' spiritual beliefs are right or wrong. We have spiritual beliefs of our own, but we do not assess the health or harm of our clients' spirituality by comparing what they believe to what we believe. What we assess is the difference that clients' beliefs make in their lives— and not just their beliefs, but also their spiritual practices, their values, and their involvement with a spiritual community.

This is a pragmatic, proof-is-in-the-pudding approach. Does a person's spirituality help her make sense of a complicated world? Does it increase her sense of agency? Does it help her treat herself and other people fairly? Does it give her life a sense of purpose and meaning? If so, then let's call it healthy. Does it make her more fearful, more agitated, or more hostile? Does it isolate her from others or from parts of herself? Does it confuse her or weaken her experience of agency? Let's call that harmful.[3]

So let's talk more about what makes spirituality healthy or unhealthy. As I've done throughout this book, I'll give you enough to get you started, but I'll be synthesizing and condensing a lot. The sources I'm synthesizing are many—family, friends, faith communities, teachers, students, mentors, writers—but the person who has sharpened my thinking most on this matter is James Griffith, particularly his book *Religion That Heals, Religion That Harms*. After you read this chapter, I strongly encourage you to read Griffith's work and go deeper.

HEALTHY AND HARMFUL
SPIRITUALITY AND RELIGION

Let's begin by considering the characteristics of harmful spirituality and religion. It's easier to do this in contrast with healthy spirituality, so we'll go there first.

Healthy spirituality and religion provide:

Deeper access to our humanness. They expand our capacity to live and feel the full range of human experience. Spirituality and religion often point beyond the human experience, of course, to a realm of transcendence. But in healthy spirituality and religion, experiences of transcendence help connect us[4] more completely to the real-deal truths of the human condition: love, loss, limits, desire, pleasure, pain, wonder, fear, gratitude, guilt, sorrow, joy, anger, helplessness, and the like.

A sense of identity. Healthy spirituality and religion help us know who we are and what is most important about us. We're in so many different roles, with so many different stressors. Healthy spirituality and religion help us get our bearings in a confusing world. Usually they point us beyond the more limited features of our identity—race, gender, nationality, and the like—to some expansive spiritual feature. They help us know who we are and what is most important about us. "I am Truth," wrote the Sufi teacher Mansur al-Hallaj (858–922). "There is nothing wrapped in my turban but God. There is nothing in my cloak but God."[5] And the New Testament writer Paul says, "It is no longer I who live, but Christ who lives in me."[6]

Connection and belonging. Healthy spirituality and religion usually connect us to a community of others who believe and practice as we do. We are part of a tribe, a family of sisters and brothers who share life with one another. We participate in rituals together—meditating, singing, blessing children, burying the dead. We share sacred texts in common, speak a special language with one another, perhaps wear distinctive clothes, and perform acts of service alongside one another. These shared experiences connect us with one another. We are not isolated and alone, but part of a group that provides social support.

A sense of worth or value. Healthy spirituality and religion bestow a sense of esteem and dignity. They say, "You matter, and here's why. This is what's important about you." But healthy spirituality and religion do not make us spiritual narcissists. They affirm the sacred worth and value of everyone and everything. "It's not just you that matters. Everything, and everyone, matters."

Comfort, strength, or meaning when we face suffering. Healthy spirituality and religion help people cope with the sorrow and pain of life. They help us make sense of suffering and are a resource for moving forward after trauma and loss. Healthy spirituality and religion do not answer all our questions about why bad things happen, but they provide at least some structure of meaning and some degree of solace and fortitude.

Support for positive character traits and secure attachment. Healthy spirituality and religion increase people's supply of wisdom, courage, kindness, humility, gratitude, self-control, and many other virtues.[7] Additionally, for people who believe in a God who wants good for them and is available to them, their relationship with God can shape and reinforce a secure attachment style.

Compassion and empathy. We are wired for empathy and compassion, and healthy spirituality and religion help increase these natural capacities in us. They help us relate with kindness to ourselves and to others. Perhaps the most distinctive mark of healthy spirituality is the way it helps us recognize the humanity of people who are not of our tribe. It helps us love our enemies.

A moral compass. Healthy spirituality and religion guide us as we navigate complex moral choices. Sometimes they might tell us exactly what to do in a difficult circumstance. ("Thou shalt not kill."[8]) Other times they offer guiding principles but leave the details up to us. ("Do justice, love mercy, walk humbly."[9]) But healthy spirituality and religion help us live ethically and with consideration for the well-being of all persons and all other creatures.

In contrast, *harmful spirituality and religion*:

Make us less human and less whole. We deny, avoid, or suppress some feature of our humanness. Some spiritualities encourage people to ignore their bodies or to see their bodies as evil. Others emphasize virtues like kindness and trust in a way that leaves people no room to acknowledge other real human feelings like anger or fear. Or they emphasize nonattachment in a way that leads people to dissociate from normal wants and desires. The result is people who become smaller versions of themselves, not their larger, more whole, more alive selves.

Make our sense of identity confused, small, or separatist. Our spiritual identity can get conflated with other features of our identity, as when "being Christian" becomes synonymous with "being American." Or we can get focused on a few beliefs, values, or practices but lose the big-picture spirit of our spiritual tradition.[10] Spirituality and religion also become unhealthy or harmful when, for the sake of fortifying our spiritual identity or the connectedness of the tribe, the line between "us" and "them" becomes rigid, and we treat outsiders differently than we treat insiders. We might avoid them, shun them, shame them, discriminate against them, label them infidels, or even commit acts of violence against them.

Lead to isolation instead of belonging. Sometimes a religious or spiritual community might exile us for violating one of its norms. Sometimes we might exile ourselves because we no longer feel worthy. And sometimes communities ask us to cut ourselves off from other important people in our lives—family, friends, neighbors—because the community's demands for purity require separation from people who are impure. But in harmful spirituality and religion, the ties that bind are broken.

Create guilt and shame instead of worth or value. Unhealthy spirituality and religion can instill or reinforce negative beliefs about ourselves. The intent here is often to make us recognize our need for help from a higher power, but the impact can be to crush our self-esteem—which also, by the way, makes us vulnerable to predatory spiritual leaders.

Do not offer comfort, strength, agency, or meaning. They may even diminish these things, making people feel worse when they suffer—because they're told their suffering is punishment for some sin, or evidence that their meditation practice isn't sufficiently advanced—or adopt a passive, powerless approach to their lives—because God is in control of everything anyway.

Diminish positive character traits and contribute to insecure attachment styles. Unhealthy spirituality and religion can reduce the degree of hope, joy, purpose, endurance, and meaning we experience. They can make us so focused on doing what's right and avoiding what's wrong that we become a ball of nerves. They can also fill us with pictures of God as threatening or distant, or whose love is conditional, thus contributing to anxious, avoidant, and disorganized attachment styles.

Engender judgment and hatred instead of compassion and empathy. Unhealthy spirituality and religion can make us critical and hostile toward ourselves or toward others, particularly others who do not believe, live, or look like we do. They can provide justification and fuel for acts of discrimination, hatred, and violence. They can be used as rationale for a variety of -isms: racism, sexism, nationalism, and so on—and become tools of interpersonal or political power.

Make people less moral. In addition to making us more hateful or aggressive, unhealthy spirituality and religion can affect our moral character in more passive ways as well. Sometimes unhealthy spirituality and religion can discourage people from seeking medical care or psychotherapeutic care.[11] Other times, they might lead us to excuse or overlook wrongs being done, to us or to others, because our religious leaders endorse what is happening or are silent about it. This is the religion Marx denounced as "opiate of the masses."[12] Otherwise moral, religious people have remained passive and idle while black people were held as slaves in the United States, while Jewish people were murdered in Nazi Germany, while global economic resources are increasingly divided unequally, and while the earth warms in a way that will be disastrous for our children and grandchildren. And while we shouldn't blame religion for all this moral passivity, we also can't ignore its contribution to it.

What you've just read is a condensed version of what could fill several books. Here's an even more condensed version. Unhealthy spirituality and religion turn people into smaller versions of themselves: less human, less at peace, less connected, less kind, less courageous, less meaning-filled, less clear about who they are and what they're about.

HOW HARMFUL SPIRITUALITY
AND RELIGION HAPPEN

Now let's talk about how this happens.

Most human beings have a twin set of needs that are somewhat in tension with each other: the need to be part of a group and the need to be an individual. Being part of a tribe—a family, a community, a team, a political group, a religion, and so on—helps us feel a sense of identity, belonging, and esteem. It also provides us moral guidance and, if it is a spiritual tribe, orientation to the realm of spiritual reality. But we also need to be seen, known, and valued as individuals. We need affirmation of our unique gifts and care for our unique challenges and hurts. And these individual needs cannot always be met at the tribal level.

Healthy spirituality and religion address and balance these two needs, but in harmful spirituality and religion, this balance is lost. Most often, the balance gets lost when the tribal functions of religion become overly strong and the needs of individuals are being neglected or abused.

To say it more pointedly: spirituality and religion become harmful when religion, the social force, causes constriction of spirituality, the personal force.[13]

Understanding how this happens is clinically quite important, so let me try to explain. First, recall the definitions of spirituality and religion I gave in chapter 4. Spirituality is all the ways you and God relate to one another, and religion is the shared beliefs, values, and practices of a group of people. There's overlap between them, but spirituality refers more to the personal, inward experience of an individual, and religion more to the shared, social experience of a group. At its best, religion, the tribal experience, serves the cause of spirituality, the personal experience. It reconnects us with God and with everything made sacred by God, including our true selves. At its worst, though, religion disconnects us and becomes a barrier to God.

The tribal function of religion is important. It's the means by which religion provides a sense of identity, belonging, and value. And to fulfill this function, to be a tribe at all, religions have to identify beliefs and behaviors that distinguish those inside the tribe from those outside. Inside the tribe, members believe certain things, practice rituals in a particular way, use language and possibly even dress in a way that is unique to them, live by a set of shared values, and relate to one another according to some spiritually sanctioned guidelines and hierarchies. The differentness is what gives insiders an identity and strengthens their sense of value and belonging. Fair enough.

But when what's required to maintain the collective strength of the tribe makes people indifferent to the needs of individuals and strangles their innate capacities for empathy and compassion, that's when religion becomes unhealthy or harmful.

Healthy religious tribes maintain a balance between the needs of the group and the needs of individuals. Healthy religion provides enough "us-ness" that we experience an orienting identity amid the disorienting chaos of the world, but not so much us-ness that we lose our capacity to see all people, inside and outside our religion, as people of worth and dignity. In harmful religion, the tribe's demand for loyalty to the rules of the tribe gets in the way of our being the kind of people the tribe is supposed to help us become. It dilutes the strength of our compassion—compassion for people outside the tribe, compassion for people inside, compassion even for ourselves.

An extreme example of group-need-for-identity-and-belonging overriding compassion-for-individuals is that of spiritual abuse. Spiritual abuse is "coercion and control of one individual by another in a spiritual context,"[14] and it can go unchallenged when loyalty to the group makes members blind to the innate humanity of other people.

Rich grew up in a family that attended a nondenominational Christian church. The pastor and youth leaders identified Rich as a troublemaker. They told him and his parents that he was possessed by the devil and that this evil spirit needed to be broken and driven out. Rich was beaten several times by church leaders; other times he was locked in a closet at the church for several days at a time. Rich escaped this church ten years ago when he left for college, but his parents and siblings are still members there. The pastor has instructed them to have no contact with Rich, and they do not. The church has become the subject of a criminal investigation in the past five years, and Rich has been interviewed numerous times in the investigation. Rich feels anxious almost all the time and has frequent flashbacks about what happened to him. He works a job in retail and takes classes part-time toward an MBA. He is around people a lot, and though he wants friends, he interacts with others as little as he can.

Religion can do harm in less extreme ways too.

Kelly is suffering from severe depression and anxiety. She's lonely, she has low energy, her thoughts are an endless stream of rumination, and she has great difficulty getting out of bed each morning and facing the day. She gets great feedback and is highly valued at work—she's a computer programmer—but she was recently placed on probation because of excessive tardiness. Her boss understands that Kelly is depressed, and he's sympathetic toward Kelly's struggle, but company policy is company policy. Kelly has almost no friends—just a few from church—and most days she goes to work and comes home, interacting only briefly with some of her coworkers, none of whom she really likes. They're not bad people, she says, but they're not church people. The church she attends draws a sharp line between believers and unbelievers. Her pastor teaches, "We're the children of light, and being with the children of darkness is dangerous," and instructs members to be wary of associating with "children of darkness." Kelly thinks it's best that she keeps to herself at work.

The teaching to beware the children of darkness is keeping Kelly from connection and friendship that would likely help her feel less depressed and anxious. Again, religion as social force, providing a sense of identity and belonging, has superseded spirituality as humanizing force.

WAKING THE INNER REFORMER

Here is the main thing to understand: religion becomes harmful when the tribal elements of religion become more influential than the inward elements of personal spiritual experience. The interventions we make follow from this understanding: the best way to intervene with harmful religion is with spirituality itself.

Let's talk about how to do that, and first, let's be clear what we don't do. We do not try to talk people out of their religious beliefs, values, or practices, or in any other way impose our own spirituality. For one thing, it's not ethical. For another, it doesn't work. Pressure from someone outside the tribe usually fortifies the resolve of those inside the tribe, and any attempt to do that—to reason, persuade, or argue—is likely to strengthen our clients' commitment when our intent is to soften it.

What does help, at least some of the time—and *nothing* works all of the time—is helping clients have an authentic spiritual experience that softens the impact of harmful religion. James Griffith puts it this way: "A clinician's prime directive is to help a patient *reassert the influence of personal spirituality* within religious life, balancing religion's valid role for creating strong social structures with empathy, compassion for self and others, whether inside or outside one's own religious group."[15] And here's the cool part: the kernel of that authentic spiritual experience is usually available right there within the harmful religion. In every religious belief and practice, even those that have become hardened, hateful, and harmful, there remains some seed of spiritual wisdom and goodness that, if contacted and nourished, can grow, bear good fruit, and create transformation.

My shorthand phrase for this intervention—for reasserting the influence of personal spirituality from inside the harmful religious frame—is "waking the inner reformer."

Here's what I mean. There is a cycle that repeats again and again in the history of religions. Religions begin when a person has a transformational spiritual experience: Buddha sitting down beneath the bodhi tree and waking up; Jesus getting baptized and hearing God say, "You are my Beloved"; Muhammad hearing the angel Gabriel in a cave near Mecca.

The reformer then talks about these experiences or lives in such a way that other people are drawn to him,[16] want to learn from him, and want to live as he lives. He shares his ideas and practices with followers, and these followers pass along stories about the teacher, repeat instructions from the teacher, and develop rituals and other practices that reinforce the way of the teacher. Thus, the original spiritual experience becomes the foundation for an organized (and sometimes codified) religion.

The *transformational* spiritual experience of an individual has now become a *formational* community. And for a while, the beliefs, values, and practices of this religious community sustain its members, animate them, move them to do good in the world, and give rise to further spiritual experiences.

Predictably, though, the religion itself becomes more important than the way of life it is meant to support. Religious practices become ends in themselves. They become rote, things people do by habit more than by heart. The container becomes more important than what it contains, the wineskin more important than the wine.[17] Religion then becomes more about morality, dogma, and group identity than about the transformation of individuals and communities. This is when it takes on all those unhealthy qualities described above.

At this point a reformer (often called a heretic) emerges, with a fresh spiritual experience. The fresh experience inspires and revives others. And there begins a new religion (or a reformation or renewal within an existing religion). The Buddha was a reformer within the Vedic traditions of India. The Hebrew prophets and Jesus were reformers within Judaism. St. Francis was a reformer within Christianity. Lao Tzu and Chuang Tzu were reformers within Confucianism.

The cyclical relationship between spirituality and religion—transformation, formation, reformation—doesn't just happen at the level of history and culture. This is how it often works clinically too. The religion in our clients' lives has become constrictive, oppressive, or numbing, but inside our clients and inside their harmful religion, there still lives an inner reformer, just waiting for someone to notice it, nourish it, and release its power to repair and renew. We are not in charge of what that inner reformer looks like or sounds like. It will wear the clothes and speak the language of our client's spiritual perspective, not ours. But the way to intervene with harmful religion without imposing our own agenda is to work within our client's unhealthy religious perspective and help that inner reformer to awaken. The way to subvert harmful religion is to help our clients connect with personal, authentic, transformational spiritual experience.

Here are six concrete clinical strategies for waking the inner reformer and helping spirituality bring healing to harmful religion.

1. Safety first
2. Use of self
3. Reinforcing healthy spirituality
4. Respectful, noncoercive inquiry
5. Referral to trusted leaders within the client's religious community
6. Naming alternative beliefs and practices

Safety First

In therapy we move at the speed of trust. Our client's trust in us and in the process of therapy is always important, but it's especially important when we're working with harmful religion. It's also especially difficult because persons affected by harmful religion are often suspicious of therapists and others outside the tribe. As a result, it's incumbent upon us to do what we can to help our clients feel safe with us and with what's happening in our office.

We promote trust and safety for our clients by meeting them with respect, empathy, and curiosity.[18] We can't fake any of these things. They're either real in us or they're not. Our clients' emotional brains are constantly tracking us—our words, our tone of voice, and our body language—to determine whether they're safe with us or not.

And we're tracking our clients too. We can't make any other interventions until they trust us, and so we watch their bodies and listen to their tone of voice for clues as to whether they're feeling safe. Are they making eye contact, or is their gaze averted? Is their posture open or closed? Is their musculature relaxed or tense? Is their tone of voice smooth or tight? Is their breathing deep and smooth or shallow and irregular?

We use words too, of course. And the words we use also help our clients know whether we respect and care for them enough for them to trust us with their spiritual experience. James Griffith recommends that we ask our clients direct questions about how their personal spiritual experience connects with the work they are doing in therapy. Here are some of his suggestions, worded for a client who uses God-talk:

- How do you feel about the therapy we're doing [or might do]? Do you have a sense that what we're doing here is in alignment with or out of alignment with God's will [or God's work] in your life?
- Do you sense that God has hopes for what happens for you in this therapy?
- In addition to this therapy, what else are you doing in your spiritual life that supports your health and healing?
- I know that you are working on this problem in different ways, and that therapy is only one of them. Help me understand how therapy fits with the larger plan.[19]

You'll want to find your own way to ask these questions, so that they'll feel real to you and your clients. But I bet you can feel the respect in those questions, and your client will too.

Use of Self

This second strategy is an extension of the first. Not only do we use our selves, particularly our embodied, nonverbal selves, to help our clients feel safe, as I have just described. We use our selves in another way too. Spiritual health is contagious, and we also use our spiritually healthy selves to infect our clients with germs of spiritual recovery. Once again, James Griffith:

> As an outgroup member, a clinician often has limited influence with members of cohesive religious groups. A respectful but persistent whole-person relatedness extended toward a patient with rigid group boundaries is perhaps the most potent of clinical interventions. Responding to another person as someone capable of reflection, empathy, concern, and compassion *tends to recruit the same processes within the other person*, while tempering activation of defensive sociobiological systems.[20]

Telling our clients "You know, you should consider being less judgmental and more compassionate" is not likely to help them become less judgmental and more compassionate. But if we embody those qualities, if that's the way we relate to them, then our clients might begin to mimic us, the way one tuning fork begins to mimic another.

There's also this benefit: by having a relationship with us, our clients are having a relationship with a person who is not of their tribe, an outsider who is, hopefully, not such a bad person after all. That experience alone often helps things begin to shift for our clients.

Reinforcing Healthy Spirituality

This third strategy is perhaps the simplest: watch for evidence of healthy spirituality in your client and offer positive reinforcement. No one is ever completely unhealthy in a spiritual sense. People who are using religion as a weapon against others or against themselves, and people having trouble setting boundaries when religion is being used as a weapon against them, are probably still doing something that we'd consider spiritually healthy. We want to catch them in the act of doing something healthy and reinforce it. In this sense, it's not that we're waking the reformer—it's already awake. We're just bringing it a cup of hot coffee and some toast with jam.

What we're looking for, to affirm and reinforce, are any behaviors that approximates spiritual wellness. These could be:

- Positive spiritual emotions, like gratitude, humility, joy, hope, and courage
- Expressions of kindness to self or others, even if those acts of kindness are limited to members of their tribe
- Personal encounters with the sacred
- Moral reasoning or moral choices that demonstrate valuing self and others

Any of these, even the smallest remnant of one of them, is a resource to be affirmed and, if possible, deepened. We do this in a number of ways. First, we mirror it. We make simple, verbal contact with it: "You felt a lot of compassion for him." "You're feeling so grateful about this." "That sounds like a God-moment."

Then maybe we bring in the basic "Tell me more about that." Or, if we think our client is up to it, we try to magnify the experience with questions like these:

- When you're feeling grateful like this, what do you notice happening physically? What does it feel like in your body?
- When you're feeling grateful like this, what thoughts go with this feeling? What do you hear yourself thinking— about God, about yourself, about other people?
- When you're feeling grateful like this, what other moments in your life does it remind you of?

Think of a set of scales. All the harmful aspects of our client's harmful spirituality are on one side; all the healthy aspects are on the other. One of the ways to counter the impact of harmful spirituality is to see how heavy we can make the healthy side.

Respectful Inquiry

The strategies we've covered thus far are mostly nonintrusive and nonchallenging. (I add "mostly" because respect, curiosity, and empathy are not completely nonintrusive. Everything we say to a client and all the nonverbal signals we send are technically intrusions—friendly intrusions, but intrusions all the same.) At times, however, we will want to enter the client's inner world more directly and stimulate the client system more actively, and the strategies we'll cover from here forward are more active in nature. If the immediately previous strategy—reinforcing healthy spirituality when it arises on its own—is like waiting attentively for the inner reformer to awaken and then bringing it coffee and toast, the following strategies are like making noise in the reformer's sleeping presence and hoping it might gently stir.

One way to gently wake the inner reformer is to ask respectful but direct and strategic questions about the harmful beliefs or practices. We don't label the belief or practice as harmful—"Can I ask you more about these unhealthy parts of your religion?"—or ask clients to explain them to us. Instead, we ask them to tell us about experiences or relationships connected to the belief or practice. For example:

- What are some times when this belief became really important to you?
- Who are some of the people you trust who helped this belief grow strong in you?
- What are some of the ways this belief has helped you live your life and relate to others in a way that you feel good about?

Notice that we ask *who* and *what* questions, not *why* questions. Why questions tend to put people on the defensive. They also direct people to their heads, which is where the rationale for the harmful spirituality lives. We want to direct people to their hearts, where memories of healthy spiritual experiences still reside, even if they're sleeping.

Whatever clients might tell us in response to our questions, we then want to validate the step of trust they've taken—"I really appreciate you telling me about this"—and do what we can to extend the conversation a little further: "Would you tell me more about that time in your life? What else was happening then?" "Would you tell me more about this person? What else stands out to you about her?"

By asking for stories about important experiences and important relationships, we are hoping to reconnect our clients with some moment of personal spiritual vitality. All the while, we're listening for the positive intention embedded in the client's harmful belief or practice—which often involves the client's need for identity or belonging—and validating that too, if we can.

Sometimes, when we ask about what has made a belief or practice so important, what we hear back is something about a passage of Scripture. And here we must acknowledge that the Scriptures of all major religions can be used to support behavior we find offensive and the law considers criminal. In every major religion, there are texts that endorse sexism and slavery,[21] and the Scriptures of Judaism, Christianity, and Islam contain texts that justify violence and genocide. To be fair, the Scriptures of every major religion also include passages that oppose these inhumane practices. But as therapists, some of the time, our clients are going to tell us that the reason they believe this, or the reason they do that, is that the Scripture says so.

We will get nowhere, of course, if we directly challenge our clients' interpretation of Scripture. The best we can do here is to ask—with great respect—about alternative perspectives within that same Scripture. Every religion has multiple viewpoints about what is true and how people are to live. If we think our client trusts us, we can ask about "minority reports" the client might be aware of.

- Are there passages of Scripture that address this in a slightly different light?
- Are there other perspectives in your religion about this matter?
- Are there times when you think about this in a different way? [Or: have there ever been times when you have thought about this in a different way?]
- I know this passage where Jesus says that adultery is the only legitimate reason for divorce is important to how you're thinking about this. Are there other words of Jesus, or stories about Jesus, that you also think about as you're trying to figure this out?
- Are there people in your church, or other people you trust, who have a different perspective?

It is almost always best to draw upon the authority of the client's religious tradition itself, not upon some authority outside their tradition. Again, most all religious traditions have plenty of health-making seeds embedded within, ready for the sunshine and water of attention and encouragement. The road to therapeutic change is paved with respectful inquiry within the client's religious frame.

Referral

If we think a belief or practice is harming our client but we don't think it's wise for us to ask a lot about it, even with respectful inquiry, another option is to try connecting that person with a wisdom figure within his religious community. Even in what appear to be unhealthy religious groups, there are often persons of spiritual maturity, wisdom, and compassion. And if there's no one trustworthy inside the client's particular community, there might be someone else they know and respect—from work, from their neighborhood, or through a common friend—who could add some perspective on what's hurting them. Referring our clients to authority figures within their religion doesn't mean we stop working with them—just that we look for help from other resources too. So we might ask, "Is there someone you really respect who you think has struggled with this, who you might feel OK asking how they've dealt with it—even how they've used their faith to deal with it?"

I asked this question of Gary, a client of mine who'd had an affair and whose guilt feelings were exacerbated by OCD and by the teachings of his church. He and I had had several conversations about guilt and forgiveness—what he believed, what Scripture had to say, what he heard about it in church—but he continued to be plagued by the idea that God's forgiveness could be conditional. So I asked if he knew someone from church with whom he could talk about guilt and forgiveness. (I'd thought that, even though Gary understood his pastor to be saying that God could withdraw forgiveness, maybe that's not what the pastor meant, and a conversation could clarify that.) But Gary said no, he wouldn't feel comfortable talking with his pastor about the affair he'd had. I then asked if he'd be open to talking to a pastor from another church, someone I knew and trusted (and whom I knew to be religiously conservative, as Gary was), but that Gary wouldn't have to face every week. Gary said yes to this offer, and this pastor was able to talk about forgiveness in a way that has helped Gary feel somewhat better.

Naming Alternate Beliefs or Practices

When our clients feel a high degree of trust with us, sometimes we can be the ones to voice a different point of view. This is the most active of the six strategies, and we would attempt this only after we are sure the client knows we have heard them, respect them, and understand their reasons for believing or acting as they do. But then we might offer the following:

- Some people [or some Christians] see it differently than that. Would you be open to hearing a different view?
- I totally understand how you feel about this, and what's led you to feel this way. I'm at a different place with it, and I wonder if you'd be willing to hear how I feel about it.

The point here is not to force a different viewpoint upon them, but to give them an experience of being safely and respectfully connected with someone who sees the world differently. Some of the examples in the last chapter, about working with spiritual struggles also illustrate this strategy.

LIVING WITH LIMITS

I've now described six respectful and noncoercive strategies for working with harmful religion. Sometimes we can use these strategies to help people recover the goodness and wisdom of personal spirituality embedded within their harm-causing religion, but sometimes we can't. Sometimes the constriction of the harmful religious perspective is just not ready to soften, and trying to force a change that's not ready to happen will most likely reinforce and strengthen the unhealthy behavior. So to the three qualities we mentioned earlier—respect, empathy, and curiosity—let's add a fourth: humility. Sometimes the best we can do, to borrow from the Serenity Prayer, is accept the things we cannot change.

CLINICAL ILLUSTRATION

I'd now like to demonstrate some of these strategies with a clinical example.

Angela came to therapy asking for help with her daughter, Kate. They have had a strained relationship for over twenty years, ever since Kate left for college. There are several reasons for the tension between them, but the one that bothers Angela most is Kate's "apostasy." Angela attends a Lutheran church, and Kate stopped going to church when she left for college. In recent years, Kate has participated in rituals with a local Wiccan community, and six months ago, when Kate's daughter, Mary Kathryn, had her first period, Kate and several of her friends held a pagan ritual to commemorate this transition. Kate invited her mother to attend, but Angela refused. It was then that Angela decided she needed to take a stand and send a clear message to Kate and Mary Kathryn about what's right and what's wrong. She wrote them a letter and told them she would no longer be part of their lives until Kate turned herself around spiritually. Kate wrote to Angela and tried calling several times, but Angela said she was not going to respond until Kate sent a clear signal that she had returned to the faith.

I had seen Angela for therapy several years before this situation, after the sudden death of her second husband, Bill. The fact that she called me for help this time suggested there was already some trust between us. But even so, it was still important that I attend to issues of safety at this tender time in her life. During her first two visits with me, she did a lot of ranting, and I did a lot of mirroring: "This is so hard." "This is agony for you." "This ritual with Kate really crossed a line for you." "You feel so disheartened." I also brought lots of curiosity to her experience: "What's the hardest part about this for you?" "How else is this affecting you?" "How is all this affecting your relationship with God?" . . . "How is this affecting the way you feel about yourself?" And of course, I asked what she wanted—"Right now, what are you hoping for? What are you wanting to happen?"—but Angela was too upset to have much clarity about those questions.

She arrived at her third session in a visibly better mood. "Something's different about you today," I said. "What's happened?" She told me she had just left a meeting at her church. She and another member were organizing a winter coat drive for children in low-income families, and they already had pledges that would buy over a hundred new coats. This sounded like healthy spirituality in action to me, so I moved to reinforce it and add weight to that side of the scale. I asked her to tell me more about it, which she did. And then I asked what made this particular project mean so much to her.

Angela: You remember that I went through a pretty ugly divorce from their father when Kate and Blake [Kate's older brother] were very young. It was all I could do to make ends meet month to month, and since I had a boy and a girl, there were no hand-me-downs. I had to buy new clothes for both of them every year. And right when they'd need their winter coats, it would also be Christmas. There were always groups that would help buy Christmas, but getting them coats was hard. I'd go to Goodwill and could always find something, but I always felt bad that they were wearing used coats.

Russell: Wow. This is really personal for you. You feel for those kids and those parents.

Angela: I really do.

Russell: And I'm so glad you've found this way to do something that's so good and that you feel so good about.

Angela: Yes.

Russell: So could I ask you another question about this? [The inner reformer is awake in her, and I'm wondering if we can deepen her connection with it.]

Angela: Sure.

Russell: Well, the fact that you're doing this, I'm wondering what it says about you, what it means about who you are as a person and a person of faith.

Angela: It doesn't say anything about me. It says something about God. I'm just a sinner. Jesus said, "I was naked and you clothed me," and he's the one who's blessed me and put me in this position to help. So this is all about him, not me.

Russell: I got it. What you're doing says something about God, not you.

Angela: That's right.

Russell: OK. [Pause] But there's still a little bit of you in this, right? You're someone who wants to do what God wants you to do. *[Here I'm offering an alternate belief for her to consider.]*

Angela: Well, that's true.

Russell: There's something in you that, at least sometimes, is able to say yes to God. *[At this point, Angela has a reflective look on her face, and I ask her what is happening.]*

Angela: I don't know. [Pause] Something is, but I don't know what it is. [Pause] And don't push me. [She smiles.] I need to let this percolate.

Russell: [I smile back.] Sounds good. I won't push. Just let it happen.

I didn't know what was happening here either, and when I asked her about it during the next appointment, she was still unable to say what it was. All she said was, "God was doing something with me that I still don't understand." I didn't know where this was heading, but I wondered if the inner reformer was awake in her and if she was having a personal spiritual experience that might soften the religious rigidity keeping her from her loved ones.

Over the next few weeks, Angela continued to hold a hard line with Kate and had no contact with her or Mary Kathryn. But her overall level of emotional distress was lower, and I used this window of calm to try developing a clearer therapeutic contract. In her first few sessions, when I asked her what she wanted, she had said, "I want Kate and Mary Kathryn back in church." This was not a goal we could work on in therapy, since neither of us had control over them, but I did not challenge her on this, since she was so upset. Now that Angela was more regulated, though, I invited her to sharpen this goal. "I want them to know right from wrong," she said, and I pointed out that this also was an outcome outside her control. "What would *you* like to be able to do?" I asked. "How would you like to be able to be in relation to them, that might in some way affect them and help them know right from wrong?"

"I want to set the right example," she told me, and then launched into a brief rant about people who claim to be Christians but don't live like Christians—Christians who believe abortion is OK and being gay is OK and that there's no consequence for sin. I wondered if my confrontation about the limits of her control, gentle as it was, had triggered this need to vent. I also recognized that the content of the vent voiced some of the unifying beliefs of her religious tribe—rallying cries—and hypothesized that she was bringing the tribe into the therapy space with her, for support, because she was emotionally distressed—about the rupture in her relationship with Kate, about the limits of her power to change Kate, and about having a therapist that was telling her, in so many words, that she wasn't in charge of other people.

These eruptions of emotional distress happen frequently in therapy, especially when we're inviting people to stretch their thinking or behavior in some way. It doesn't mean we've done something wrong—it's our job to help people stretch—but it does mean we might need to slow down and shore up the client's experience of trust. Safety first!

It actually did not take long—just a few minutes of mirroring, with a soothing voice—before her face and tone of voice signaled that she was emotionally regulated again. Then she was the one to pick back up the thread of our conversation.

Angela: I do want to set the right example. I really do.

Russell: That sounds really, really important to you.

Angela: It is. Very important.

Russell: Can I ask you more about that? [She nods yes.] Like . . . how . . . how did setting the right example, for her and for others, get to be as important to you as it is? Or maybe . . . who did that for you? Who set a right example for you? Or was there a time in your life where it really got clear to you how important that is? [I'm hoping that respectful inquiry might evoke a memory that gets inside the religious rigidity and connects her to a personal spiritual impulse.]

Angela: You ask hard questions!

Russell: I know. I know. But you ask hard questions too! [We laugh.] But seriously, this is at the heart of all this for you—setting a good example for Kate and Mary Kathryn—and I'd like to know how it got to be as important to you as it is.

Angela: Well, I never told you this about Bill [her deceased husband], but he and I didn't get together in the most moral of circumstances. [She raises her eyebrows, as if asking me to read between the lines.]

Russell: I think I understand.

Angela: And there was a lot of judgment, and I didn't feel like I could go to church anymore. And I had Kate and Blake with me only every other week. And it was just a hard time, a time I'm not proud of. . . . I'm proud of the way I kept going. But I'm not proud of how Bill and I got together, even though it was another five years before we totally went public with our relationship and got married. And eventually Kate and Blake found out, when they were older. . . . Anyway, do you understand what I'm trying to say?

Russell: I might, but I'm not sure.

Angela: I'm saying I wasn't always the best example to my kids, and I can't help but think if I'd been a stronger Christian when I was younger, and kept those kids in church, maybe Kate's life would have been different.

Russell: OK, now I understand. Maybe. Are you saying you feel . . . responsible? For Kate?

Angela: Yes. I do. I *am* responsible. And that's why I'm determined to set a better example now. For her and for Mary Kathryn.

Russell: Wow. I get it. That really helps. You really love her, and you feel like you failed her when she was younger. And you're trying to set a right example now.

Angela: That's right.

Russell: So I bet you know what I want to ask you now.

Angela: Probably another hard question.

Russell: Probably so. Let's find out. What I'm wondering about is what it means to you to set a right example. That can mean so many things, you know? So for you, from the perspective of your faith, what are the different things that means? [*My thinking here is that Angela has been locked in on one meaning of "right example"—being loyal to the one true faith—and the words I'm choosing here—"many things," "different things"—are subtle attempts to help her consider alternate perspectives within her own faith.*]

Angela:	Well, the example I want to set is to point the way to Christ.
Russell:	You want your example to point them to Christ.
Angela:	Yes.
Russell:	Right, but I'm wondering: what are the different ways you do that? . . . Are doing that? . . . Want to do that?
Angela:	Well, I've told Kate, very clearly, that all this Wiccan stuff is of the devil, and that she's playing with fire. And I've set a firm limit, that as long she's involved with all that, there's just no point in us having a relationship.
Russell:	So you're setting an example with your words, telling her clearly what you believe, and also with your actions, by refusing to see her and talk with her because of this.
Angela:	That's right.
Russell:	So now I'm wondering . . . and let me give you a little warning, this might be another hard question, but I think you know I'm trying to help you, right?
Angela:	I do.
Russell:	And I know this is agony for you, seeing Kate be apart from the faith, and being cut off from her and Mary Kathryn. . . . Anyway, my question is: What else does your faith have to say about setting

an example for other people? Besides an example of belief, besides an example of setting limits at certain times, are there other perspectives, maybe even other parts of Scripture, that speak to you about this?

Angela: [She sighs.] I'll need to pray about that.
Russell: All right.

Angela was still committed to the no-contact-until-you've-changed boundary with her daughter and granddaughter, but several important things were happening. We had a more workable therapeutic contract: helping her set a right example. We had learned that the impetus for this goal was partly related to her religious beliefs and partly related to an emotional burden she was carrying: guilt about her long-ago affair and not setting the kind of example for her kids she would have wanted. We had also learned that she, who was now using her spirituality in a rather harsh way, had herself been on the receiving end of spirituality used harshly. And we had opened up space for additional insights about setting a right example to emerge from within her spiritual framework. The inner reformer was at work, and we were clearing space for it to continue.

Over the next month, Angela immersed herself in Bible study and prayer. She asked God to show her what it meant to set a right example for Kate and Mary Kathryn, and a big shift happened when she read a verse in the New Testament about "speaking the truth in love."[22] "I know I'm speaking the truth," she told me. "There's only one way to the Father, and that's through the Son, not through all this Wiccan stuff. But I have to admit that I'm not speaking that truth in a loving way. And that's not the example I want to be setting."

And this, you recognize, was a turning point—a turn brought about not by my imposing my beliefs and values on her, but by my helping her engage her own beliefs and values more deeply.

There was not a straight line from that turning point to a reopening of relationship with her daughter and granddaughter. Angela experienced a lot of back-and-forth internally. Part of her felt that swallowing her pride and reconnecting with them was the right thing to do, but part of her worried that a shift on her part would be misinterpreted as a concession on the matter of belief. We continued work to deepen her own acceptance of forgiveness and to experience recovery from the spiritual injury she had experienced when being shunned by her church years ago.

Eventually, Angela chose to write a letter to Kate, and she asked me to help her work on it. The letter became something of a mirror in which Angela could see her anguish and bitterness, and in her sessions, we would work on the emotional and spiritual blockages the letter-writing revealed. It took six weeks for her to complete it, but it represented her well. She apologized for having cut off connection, named that their spiritual differences were still difficult for her but that being apart from Kate and Mary Kathryn was even more difficult, and asked if Kate would be willing to give them a chance to reconnect.

The story of their reconnection was not a straight line either. It was as ambiguous and messy as you might expect. But I have shown you what I wanted: how Angela's faith, which was supporting the emotional hardness she felt toward her daughter, became the source of its softening—and how I, as therapist, kept alert for her inner reformer to appear and used our relationship to help it grow stronger.

CONCLUSION

Our human propensities for prejudice, anxiety, and aggression are amplified when they operate with the support of a religious rationale, and in this way, religion can do great harm in the world. But within every religion, even those that have become twisted and toxic, and within every religious person are seeds of curiosity, calmness, and kindness that can be nourished into the material and means of transformation. Harmful religion gets healed in therapy the same ways it gets healed everywhere else: via human connection, in relationships that become safe, and with respect and care for the humanness of those who are injured and those who do the injuring.

Meeting harmful religion with judgment, frustration, or force is of no use. But meeting it with kindness, humility, and truth, as well as with the therapeutic strategies described in this chapter, can be powerful medicine.

It takes a certain kind of faith to look at the obscenity and ugliness of harmful religion and believe that, somewhere in there, an inner reformer still lives, that there are seeds of transformation waiting for just the right kind of sunlight to land on them and awaken them.

A certain kind of faith is where you come in. And it is now to you, your spiritual perspective, and how you make use of it as a therapist that we turn our attention.

PART THREE

Working with
Your Own Spirituality

10

Spirituality and
Your Overall Approach
to Psychotherapy

You now have a basic framework for what's involved in working with your client's spirituality: how to enter into spiritual conversation, how to understand your client spiritually, and how to make skillful interventions.

But this is only half the story. You are not a vending machine that dispenses empirically supported interventions from some objective location swept clean of beliefs and values. You are a human being, with spiritual beliefs, values, and practices of your own, and working with spirituality in psychotherapy also includes what you do with these. It's about giving conscious consideration to how your own spiritual orientation affects your work. It's also about giving attention to the unconscious material that bubbles up moment to moment in response to your clients—the steady stream of sensation, emotion, and memory that we call *countertransference.*

The next three chapters are a brief treatment about how to do this: how to draw upon your spirituality without imposing it. In this chapter, I will make the case for why giving attention to your own spirituality is important, describe a few ways that my own spirituality affects my approach to psychotherapy in general, and invite you to consider how your spirituality affects your approach. In chapter 11, I will relate several clinical examples that illustrate how my spirituality affected my work in very specific clinical moments. And in chapter 12, I will give attention to spiritual countertransference.

In all three chapters, my hope is to expand your awareness of how your spirituality affects your work, increase the freedom you feel to let that happen, and strengthen your confidence that you're doing this in a manner that affects your work and your clients in a positive way.

OUR SPIRITUALITY IS ALWAYS PRESENT

Therapists do not usually tell clients, "Here's what I believe spiritually." For that matter, we don't usually tell them, "Here's what I believe psychologically" either. If our calling in the world is to explain psychological theory, we become a professor, and if our calling is to share our spiritual beliefs, we become a minister, imam, rabbi, or some other spiritual teacher. As therapists, our job is to help clients find their own true path, in a way that is authentic and useful to them. It's not that we never convey our own ideas to clients, but we are mindful that ideas are laden with meaning and values, and we are careful not to impose them. We're also mindful that "explaining things" can impede "experiencing things," and because we want to help our clients have new experiences, not just new thoughts, we are selective about when and how we share ideas. There are occasional exceptions to this rule, but by and large, we do not talk about our own spirituality with our clients.

That said, our own spirituality is always in the room. It is an integral part of our humanness, and like other aspects of our humanness—gender, race, social location, personality, physical appearance, life experience, and the like—it cannot be separated out from who we are and how we work. It shapes our understanding of what helps people live happy, healthy, meaningful lives. It frames our perspective on suffering. It infuses our personal presence with humility, compassion, wisdom, and other intangible qualities that help clients trust us and feel hopeful about change. And it is a resource for us, a store of kindness, clarity, and courage that helps us do the work we do.

All this to say: our own spirituality is a big part of who we are and what we do with clients, and it's important to think about what our spiritual assumptions are and how they affect our work. I want to help you do that.

HOW SPIRITUALITY AFFECTS
OUR APPROACH TO PSYCHOTHERAPY

The ideal way to help you consider how spirituality affects your practice would be in a conversation—you, me, maybe a few others, sitting outside somewhere and talking. But since we're in a book and not a backyard, we'll do it this way: I'll share some of my spiritual beliefs and describe how they affect my approach to therapy. And you, anytime you're hit with a thought about what you believe and how it affects your work, put the book down and follow that thought. Maybe take a few notes or talk it through with a friend. I'll be right here when you return.

Our interest here—the way our spirituality affects our practice—is in what we might call a "spiritual psychology." If a "psychology" is a theory that explains human consciousness and behavior, a "spiritual psychology" is a theory that explains human consciousness and behavior and that includes, or even makes central, spiritual ideas and dynamics.

All clinical psychologies, and all theories of psychotherapy, address three questions:

1. What is fundamentally true about people?
2. How do people become unhealthy?
3. How do unhealthy people get healthy again?

The first question concerns our understanding of human personality and development, the second our understanding of psychopathology, and the third our understanding of change, including how psychotherapy is part of the change process. A spiritual psychology addresses the same three questions, from a spiritual perspective, and I'll be using those questions to organize what follows.

Some of you will resonate with what I say here. Some of you won't. I offer it not as a recommendation—"My spiritual psychology is awesome! You should see things this way too!"—but as an invitation for you to be conscious and thoughtful about the spiritual beliefs that affect the way you practice.

What Is Fundamentally True about People?

I believe that what's most true about people is what's most true about everything: we are made of spiritual energy.

Science itself, since Einstein, has recognized that matter is made of energy: $e = mc^2$. I believe something more, something neither verifiable nor falsifiable: that this energy, which is the substance and structure of everything, has a spiritual quality to it. Call it whatever poetic word you want—God, Love, the Life Force, the Really Real—it is the source and substance of all that is: stars and stones, birds and bees, streams and trees (especially trees). What brings the material into being, and sustains it in its being, continuously, is spiritual energy, a vibrating energy of the kind sound makes—which is why, for me, it feels true when Genesis says the world was created by sound, the words "Let there be," or when a Hindu mystic like Yogananda says the world proceeds continuously from sound, the vibratory Aum of divine consciousness.[1]

People are made of this spiritual energy that is like sound. (The word "person," in English, comes from Old French: it means "to sound through"—*per*, through + *sonare*, to sound. Perhaps this is why music moves us so deeply: it is the language of souls and cells.) We are part of God, and God is part of us.[2] What is most true of us is that we are expressions of an Infinitely Vast Spiritual Reality that is always sounding through us, always expressing something of Itself through us, always trying to "happen" in us.

I don't say any of this to clients, mind you. But it is the behind-the-scenes, in-my-bones perspective that grounds me and affects how I understand what I'm doing as a therapist.

And what I'm doing as a therapist is, largely, just collaborating with this spiritual energy that is the most true thing about us. I am working in concert with God who is the source of truth, beauty, and goodness in all persons. I do not have to install anything essential or squeeze anything good out of my clients. I do not have to teach people where the Light is or in which direction the path to better is. These potentials are already there, part of all persons' innate connection to Divine Love. I am simply watching for them to happen, watching for my clients to do any of the things people do when God is happening in them. Then, using the "strengthening a spiritual resource" strategies described in chapter 7, I give those things my backing.

I'm watching for people to do things like:

- Feel gratitude and say "Thank you"
- Feel compassion and offer kindness, to others or to themselves
- Reach out for connection and attachment, with God, with themselves, and with others, including the therapist
- Ask for help

- Set boundaries
- Apologize
- Receive apologies and extend forgiveness
- Experience healthy dependency; feel supported; receive kindness, comfort, and nourishment
- Mobilize for action; exercise agency and power
- Slow down; come to rest; practice moments of Sabbath
- Show curiosity (the opposite of prejudice or assumption)
- Seek meaning and try to make sense of things
- Wrestle with a moral choice; try to discern right action in a complicated situation
- Demonstrate creativity, including humor
- State a desire—I want, I prefer—sometimes directly, through words, and sometimes indirectly, through the energy in their voice[3]
- State an intention—I will, I won't[4]
- Make a decision
- Have a thought and speak it
- Feel or express emotion

These are some of the ways God happens in people, and something of God is always happening in every person who comes for help. No one is ever missing the shimmer and spark of Love, no one is ever without wisdom, no one is ever beyond hope. No matter how cracked, crushed, or chaotic a person's life has become, the seeds of recovery are already sewn. My job is to collaborate with that.

How Do People Become Unhealthy?

Another thing I believe, spiritually, is that while we are made of Love and Love is always present in us, we often lose awareness of that Reality. I won't babble on here about how or why this happens, but our relationship with God gets warped or broken, and though it never stops being Really Real in us and around us, our capacity to experience God—and our relationship with God—seems to vanish. We live with an almost constant case of spiritual amnesia.[5]

In this state of spiritual amnesia, we get smaller. The world we're aware of shrinks from the size of a God to the size of an I. We stop being our God-sounding-through true self[6] and take residence in the too-small shelter of a small self, a false self,[7] what the transpersonal psychologists and others call "ego." We constrict to the size of our small self-identifications—identifications with our history, roles, relationships, and affiliations, as well as with our physical and emotional cravings—and lose awareness of the Larger Self.

I don't say any of this aloud to clients either, but these beliefs also affect my approach to therapy: the work of therapy is not just to collaborate with the healing, expansive, liberating action of Love in our clients. It is also to keep watch for its opposite—the painful, constrictive, imprisoning action of spiritual amnesia—and interrupt it.

I am on the lookout for my clients' smallness and falseness, for the trances that numb them, the attachments that confine them, and for the way these small or sleepy compulsions create misery and diminish meaning. I try to watch for these life-constricting patterns with eyes of Love, not judgment, and I invite clients' attention—also with eyes of Love—to the thoughts, feelings, physical sensations, movements, and behaviors that keep them small and bring them suffering.

Then—having watched for these patterns, reflected them back, and enlisted clients in observing them and studying them for themselves—I invite clients to stretch, to step outside their habit, to interrupt it, if only for a moment. I want to help them try something different—substitute a different thought, sit with their emotion a moment longer before speaking, relax their shoulders in the presence of this enemy—and notice what happens next.

I often tell supervisees that therapy is the same two things, over and over: noticing and interrupting. Help your clients notice the habitual patterns in their lives that aren't working (many of them unconscious), and interrupt them with some modest (but often quite courageous) experiment that alters the pattern in some way. This is how psychological change happens.

Spiritual change can also happen in this way. While spiritual change is not usually the goal of psychotherapy, noticing and interrupting sometimes helps the small self die to itself, which makes space for its rebirth as something more expansive, powerful, and true. Therapists are not pastors, and therapy is not spiritual direction. We do not impose our spiritual values or require that our conversations include explicit spiritual language. But the changes that happen on our watch do have a spiritual component, and people often have a sense that the empowering presence of Love is growing stronger in them.

How Do Unhealthy People Get Healthy Again?

In several of the paragraphs above, I said that I try to relate to my clients with an attitude of Love. These statements reflect two other of my primary spiritual beliefs: first, that the way back to health is by a reawakening to the Reality of Love (the Reality of Love that is always there but about which we have amnesia), and second, that what reawakens people to the Reality of Love is actual contact with Love.

This contact can happen any number of ways:

- Through connection with another person—a family member or friend, a stranger or an enemy, a teacher, a coach, a minister, or a therapist
- Through connection with animals—domesticated and wild
- Through other experiences with the natural world
- Through art—stories, songs, sculptures, and more

- Through religious ritual
- In moments of silence and stillness

Love—which is to say, God—is present in all things. There are bodhi trees and burning bushes everywhere.

These twin beliefs—that what helps people change is a reawakening to Love through an experience with Love—affect my approach to therapy in this manner: the most important thing I offer clients, and what helps people change, is Love. Not mindfulness, or cognitive restructuring, or motivation enhancement, or bilateral stimulation: Love.

What I'm saying here is not to dismiss the importance of psychotherapy theory and technique. I am a theory geek and a technique junkie. I have spent much time learning Internal Family Systems Therapy, Sensorimotor Psychotherapy, EMDR, and other therapeutic approaches. The perspectives and protocols of those models are extremely helpful in the work I do, and I use them all, shall we say, religiously. But apart from Love, theory and technique are clanging cymbals. What makes a difference, what changes lives, is Love.

Love is not exactly an intervention, of course. It is more a spirit that infuses the entire therapeutic frame and everything that happens within it. Love is my attitude toward my client. It is the energy that holds and empowers both of us in each moment. Love does not mean I am friends with my clients. It does not mean I don't charge a fee for my service or keep other boundaries that make therapy safe for them and for me. Love means willing good for my clients and opening my heart in their presence. It means surrendering my need for certainty and softening whatever tendencies I have for use of force. Love means allowing myself to be affected, moved—even, in some ways, hurt—by my clients. It means making my heart and myself available as a channel for the unseen energy of God.

Let me enlarge upon that last sentence and be even more personal. My experience of the "unseen energy of God" is often quite physical. Sometimes I notice it is as vibration humming throughout my body, other times as light shining on my heart, or a featherlike whisper around my skin, or the energy of an ocean moving through the single drop that is me. Paying attention to these physical sensations as they happen—being mindful of them—helps regulate my nervous system and increases my sense of peace and power. And since "the brain is a social organ,"[8] as interpersonal biology researchers have shown, it also helps regulate the nervous system of my client. Additionally, though—and here I am saying something more than interpersonal neurobiology does, something entirely unprovable—I think noticing these somatically spiritual sensations helps unleash and midwife the energy of Love more fully in the room.

Sometimes it actually feels like there is a mirror in my heart that I can adjust and use to reflect the Light of Love toward my client. Or that the flow of Love through me is something I can channel in my client's direction. And, although I may be imagining all this or projecting it, sometimes it looks to me like my clients are feeling this expanding spiritual energy and are affected by it. I do not strain to do any of this channeling or reflecting. Straining is an act of the small self and blocks the presence of Real Love. But I believe there is something about my willing participation in the presence of Love—something about the *yes* I say to it—that actually helps it happen.

It can go the other way too. My defenses, my asleepness, my fixations, compulsions, blind spots, trances, and constrictions are continually clogging the arteries of my heart and limiting the Love I'm able to channel. There are clients from whom my first impulse is to withdraw. There are other clients with whom I overidentify and to whom I am drawn too closely. There are times when I am preoccupied by some drama in my own life,

and I do not make my mind and heart available for deep listening. There are times I am afraid of a client; envious of a
client; or attracted to, hurt by, or angry with a client. There are
times when I feel tired, or believe, "I just don't have it today,"
and I resist going to the deeper places where healing is possible.
There are times when I'm trying too hard.

All of this is real, and normal, and common experience for
therapists. It is also the action of the smaller self—I say this
without any judgment, toward myself or others—and I want to
surrender the will of my smaller self to the Larger Will of Love,
for my clients' sake and for my own.

At a practical level, what this means is offering myself the
same thing I offer my clients: noticing and interrupting with
Love. I try to notice my thoughts, feelings, and actions, greet
them with kindness, learn their ways, hear what they're saying, receive their wisdom, and connect their fears and concerns
with the presence and support of Love. Love softens the constriction and urgency of my smaller self and opens my heart
more fully, so that I am as much the vessel and instrument of
Love as I can be.

CONCLUSION

There are other applications of my spirituality to the work of
therapy, but the ones I have described are enough to give you
a flavor for how spirituality informs me and, I hope, evokes
awareness of how your spirituality is informing you. Before
reading on, take a minute (or sixty) and notice some of the
ways you think your spiritual orientation affects the way you
do your work. Meditate and mull over the three questions that
all psychologies address—what's most true about people, how
do people become unhealthy, and how do they get healthy
again—and be curious about how your spirituality colors the
way you answer them.

Give your own spirituality some room to breathe in your practice. Set yourself a frame that keeps you from imposing your beliefs and values on your clients—humility helps with this—and within that safe frame, give your spirituality freedom to help you. Let it expand the range of your understanding and the depth of your presence. The quality of your work and the satisfaction you receive from it will both increase.

11

....

Spirituality and
Specific Moments in
Psychotherapy

IN THE LAST CHAPTER I ASKED YOU TO CONSIDER HOW YOUR
behind-the-scenes spiritual orientation—what you believe
about Life, Reality, God, or whatever you call it—already affects
your overall approach to psychotherapy, and could affect it even
more if you let it.

In this chapter we'll take another step, from "therapy in
general" to "therapy in particular." Here I'll provide you with
concrete clinical illustrations that show me drawing upon my
spiritual perspective, letting it influence the clinical process,
but not pushing it or imposing it on my clients. I hope that seeing this boundary in action, in real-time clinical encounters,
will strengthen your confidence that you can do the same.

I'm giving you three examples. In the first, not a single explicitly spiritual word gets spoken by me or the client,

illustrating well the way spiritual awareness and spiritual guidance can be happening in the mind and heart of the therapist, and can affect what the therapist then says and does with the client, but without the therapist ever saying anything overtly spiritual. In the other two examples, one involving a client, the other a supervisee, I do use explicit spiritual language, because that it is the language the client and supervisee use. But even here, where the client (or supervisee) and I share a common spiritual language, you'll see that I am drawing upon spiritual perspectives but not imposing them. In all three, you will notice the influence of the spiritual psychology I outlined in the previous chapter.

ENGAGE YOUR SPIRITUAL CAPACITY, PLEASE

Everyone is spiritual. I've said that throughout this book, and I believe it's true. But not everyone is connected with their spiritual capacity or making use of it. Think of the children's song, "Row, row, row your boat, gently down the stream." Everyone lives in a spiritual stream, but not everyone is rowing. When we row, especially when we row gently and not anxiously, our spiritual body is strengthened.[1] We become less constricted in our smaller selves and live more fully in our true selves. And the way to row, spiritually speaking, is by using any of our various spiritual capacities: awareness, kindness, gratitude, generosity, intention, agency, and many, many others.

Sometimes it strikes me that a client's life could be better, or symptoms reduced, if he or she did a little more rowing and strengthening of spiritual capacity. It's fun to think of creative ways to invite clients to exercise their spiritual bodies, especially when the client does not identify with an explicit spiritual tribe, does not speak a particular spiritual language, and would likely be turned off if I introduced any explicit spiritual language. This is the case in the next example. Without using any explicit spiritual language, I ask the client, in so many words, "Would you please activate your spiritual capacity?"

Amy came for therapy for help with significant mental health issues that have wrecked her life. On the phone and in her first appointment, she described a years-long struggle with bipolar disorder, PTSD, substance abuse, and legal trouble.

Amy is thirty-one, and once or twice a year, for most of the past ten years, she has had a disastrous manic episode. She gets loud, talks fast, violates other people's personal space, refuses to leave stores and restaurants, breaks things, and assaults people who challenge her, cops included. In some of these episodes she has become psychotic. She has been hospitalized six or seven times and arrested twice. After her most recent arrest and hospitalization, about three months before calling me, she moved in with her parents. She has regular conflict with them but cannot afford to pay her own rent. She works in the service industry and functions well there until she becomes manic.

She says that she has experienced trauma—as a child and as an adult—and wants to process these experiences. But at this point in our work, eight sessions in, she has not wanted to talk about those experiences, and I know few details about them. It is clear that she wants to approach these topics slowly, and I respect her sense about the pacing of our work.

She says she is spiritual but not religious, so her spiritual resources are all implicit ones: internal resources like her intelligence, sense of humor, confidence, and a certain swagger, and external resources like a strong relationship with her brother, a dog she loves, music, creative writing, exercise, and being outdoors.

In our work this far, we have focused on building tools for emotional regulation (including mindfulness), reconnecting her with a psychiatric support system, and developing strategies for working with the significant stressors in her life (work, her parents, dating).

In the session I share below, our eighth, she began by saying she has had a very bad week. She was worried about money, she has had several difficult customers at work, and she had a big argument with her mother. She was quite agitated as she reported all this. She was using more profanity than usual, and to an extent, she seemed to be enjoying herself as she talked about it. I wondered if the hypo-manic state she was in could escalate into a more severe and dangerous mania, and I decided to experiment with an intervention.

Russell: Can I pause you for a moment?

Amy: [Laughs] I'm kinda wound up, aren't I? *[This is one of those moments where I think,* It might help this person to have a bit more spiritual strength working for her, *so I ask her to build some spiritual strength by using the mindfulness skills we've worked on previously.]*

Russell: Well, you tell me. How about notice, like you've practiced here before. Notice what's happening in your thoughts and in your body, and in a minute let me know what you're aware of.

Amy: [Silence for twenty seconds] I'm aware of angry words in my head. Those things I was saying to you, that I'd said to my mom, and thought about my mom. And the things I think about rude customers. I'm still hearing those in my head. . . . And in my body . . . a lot of agitation. All over my body. But mainly in here [points to her chest].

Russell: OK. Great. And I hear . . . I don't know. . . . Right now I hear a shift in your voice. *[Again, I'm asking her to exercise her capacity for awareness, this time by mirroring back the shift in vocal tone I've noticed.]*

Amy: Yes. For sure. Definitely a shift in energy. I wish
                I could do this when I'm mad at my mom or at
                work.

Russell: OK. That's actually what I was wondering. When
                you're mad at somebody, your mom or somebody
                at work, or when your energy goes in a manic
                direction in some other situation, what would
                you like to be able to do? *[Here I'm asking her to
                exercise a slightly different spiritual capacity, that of
                setting intention.]*

Amy: I'd like to be able chill the . . . you-know-what . . .
                out.

Russell: And what would be good about that? How would
                it affect your life in a good way if you could do
                that? *[If you know Motivational Interviewing, you
                probably recognize these questions.]*

Amy: Are you kidding? I'm working for twelve dollars
                an hour. I've got a thousand dollars in court costs.
                I'm thirty-one and living with my mom and dad.
                All because of mania. All because I can't chill
                out. So it would be great if I could have more
                self-control.

Russell: But it's so fun to be manic! [We both laugh.] So
                satisfying to tell somebody off! You want to give
                that up?

Amy: Oh my God. Don't make me hit you! [Smiling]

Russell: All right, all right. So you've got these tools for
                bringing your nervous system back in balance.
                We've talked about them and practiced them
                here. You've been practicing them on your own
                too. But when you're in one of those moments—
                someone's bugging you, and your energy starts to

rise, you start telling them off in your head, and you're about to go off on them—if you could use one of these tools, maybe you wouldn't go off. Maybe you'd stay calm and handle the situation in a way you'd feel good about later. Maybe you wouldn't get arrested or end up in the hospital. But here's the thing: to do any of that, to use any of these tools you're building, there's something in you—I don't know what you'd call it—but there's some part of yourself, something deep in you, that's got to turn on. It's got to turn on to activate your good intention, your willingness to use those tools you've been working on. You know what I mean? There's got to be something in you that wants to do that. Is this making any sense? *[Here I am describing a spiritual function, as best I can, without using any explicit spiritual words. With another client, I might use the word "spirit" here, but she does not belong to a "spirit" tribe, and using that word would create a rupture and interrupt the exercise I'm inviting her to try. I am hoping to engage her curiosity about the spiritual capacity within herself. I do not care what she calls it. I simply want her to look inwardly for some "first mover" in herself. I believe that if she can notice this capacity in herself, it will strengthen it. Energy follows attention, as they say.[2] Even looking for it, whether or not she finds it, will strengthen it.]*

Amy: Yes, definitely. There's got to be something that calls me to myself.

Russell: Yeah, that's it. I wish I coulda said it like that. So, let me ask you, where is that in you? *[Here again, I am asking her to direct her attention inwardly, because I believe that looking and noticing will strengthen her spiritual capacity.]*

Amy: Where is it in me?

Russell: Uh-huh. This thing that calls you to yourself, that has to move first before any of the other things that need to happen will happen, if you're going to listen for it, or watch for it, or feel for it, or whatever—where do you direct your attention? Where inside yourself?

Amy: [Pauses, drops eyes, seems to be mindful] Um, in my heart area, and also in my face. Is that weird?

Russell: No, not at all. So maybe just stay with that for a minute, just sensing in to your heart area and your face, and let that part of you just be there, happen, do whatever it does right now.

Amy: [Silence, greater stillness of body] It's hard to describe, but it feels like something that's just behind everything else, physically behind it, I mean. . . . Something really still . . . and quiet . . . but it also has a lot of energy. Not energy. Power.

Russell: OK. And does it feel all right to be aware of it and connecting with it this way?

Amy: Definitely. It feels great.

Russell: So maybe just sit with this a little more, and let it soak into your muscle memory a bit . . . like a soft rain soaks into the earth.

Without saying explicitly, "Hey, I think your spiritual self could help you here," I invited Amy to be curious about the spiritual part of herself and to try bringing it a bit more into the present moment. Whether she ever thinks of herself as spiritual or not, I believe that using and strengthening this part of herself can lessen the power of her small self and increase the quality of her life.

MORE AGENCY, PLEASE

Now I offer an example with a client who is explicitly religious, and with whom I do intervene with religious language.

Stephen is fifty-three, a social worker, and twice divorced. Five years ago he reconnected with his high school sweetheart, Anita, and it is trouble in this relationship that brought him to therapy.

Things were great with Anita for the first six months. It was good to be in love again, and being with her, the person he had dated at age sixteen, also reconnected him with a younger version of himself. But then her drinking increased, and Anita is a volatile drunk. She would insist that he stay the night, which he would do, and then she would stay up all night, drinking, watching TV, and running the vacuum cleaner. Sometimes she hit him. If he tried to leave, to go home where he might get some sleep, she would threaten to kill herself. Gradually, over the past five years, she had become financially dependent on him: he helps her pay her mortgage some months, it's always his credit card that gets swiped at restaurants and at the grocery, and he recently cosigned for a car loan. Occasionally he confronts her about her behavior and threatens to end the relationship. But he loves her, he says; she promises she'll change; and she says the real problem isn't her, anyway. It's him. It's his weakness, she says, the way he lets other people take advantage of him, that upsets her so much. So, he stays, even though for the past four years he says he has felt like a hostage.

Stephen is "a giver." He currently works at a nursing home, and he regularly goes above and beyond what's required. He finds it depressing to be there, but old people love him, and having lost both his parents, he feels especially tender toward the patients and their families. In the spring he coaches a Little League team. He has a son from his first marriage and, through his son, a grandson. His son struggles with finances from time to time, so Stephen pays for the grandson's daycare. (This is one of the reasons for Anita's criticism.)

Stephen was raised in a stable home. His father was a Baptist minister, his mother a middle-school teacher. They expected Stephen to "be a good boy." He was, and they loved him for it. He developed a strong sense for knowing what others wanted from him and who they wanted him to be, but not so strong a sense for knowing who he is and what he wants for his life. While his parents were alive, he never risked learning whether they would still love him if he did something other than what they expected or wished for him.

This relational strategy worked well enough for him in his family of origin, but not so well in either of his marriages. Both his wives loved him at first—he was great at being attentive and kind—but over time each grew frustrated at how needy he was for affection and appreciation. Like Anita does now, they also told him he was weak, and both left him by way of affairs.

Stephen attended a Methodist church with his first wife and now attends a nondenominational Christian church. He teaches Sunday school, serves as an elder, and volunteers with the youth group. He is much loved by church members and appreciated for all he does, but he has little contact with them beyond the time he spends at church activities. Anita discourages these relationships; she says they get too much of him already.

He does not pray, he says. He believes he should and feels guilty that he doesn't, but he just never seemed to be able. For years he tried praying, but nothing ever seemed to happen, and it was hard to gather much momentum for it. Plus, he says, even when he did pray, what good did it do? It didn't seem like his life was any better for it, so a few years ago that part of his spiritual life fizzled out entirely.

Other than his parents, it seems, nobody has fully appreciated and rewarded his efforts to please—not his wives, not Anita, not even God. He knows how to make other people happy, but no one seems to know how to make him happy. On the outside, he is upbeat and positive. It's the way other people like him to be. But on the inside, he feels lonely, frustrated, and sad. He has adopted a passive, dependent approach to life, and he's not been able to muster the bravery or the will to find his voice, assert himself, and risk a degree more agency.

The session I am describing below is our twentieth. In our early sessions, I felt lots of empathy for Stephen. What a likable guy he is! And what a tough situation! But as the weeks passed, session after session of complaining without action, complaining without action, complaining without action, I grew frustrated.

Through the years I've learned to appreciate frustration when I feel it toward a client. It's almost always a reliable internal supervisor, an indicator that something needs changing in my clients' lives or in the way we're working together. I've also learned that frustration is a great supervisor but a lousy communicator. As a result, I've learned to hear its wisdom but use a different part of myself to communicate that wisdom to my clients.

In this case, my frustration was saying, "He needs to grow a spine, speak up, and take action." But he already knew that, at least at some level. The question was: What can be done about it? What might increase his capacity for agency? What might help him move from an overly passive mode into a mode where the active and receptive dimensions of his personality are in more healthy balance with one another?

One of my favorite spiritual interventions involves helping people experience their way into a healthier active-receptive balance by facilitating a conversation between them and God.[3] I think you'll get the hang of this intervention by reading the conversation below, but the gist of it is that the therapist becomes something of a couples therapist, or family therapist, between the client and God, helping the client to speak more and listen more.

Russell:	I'm wondering if, as you're going through all this, if you ever imagine God looking in, noticing, understanding. . . .
Stephen:	I really don't. I know I should.
Russell:	I'm not thinking that you should. . . . I was just wondering if you did. . . . But now that I hear you don't, it makes me wonder, how come?
Stephen:	I feel the same way about God that I do about Anita. I don't trust either of them. [He blurts this out immediately, with no pause, as if this thought had been forming, simmering, and waiting in him for a long time and was finally getting a chance to be spoken.]
Russell:	[Nods encouragingly]
Stephen:	"I'm doing so much for you, and you're not doing anything for me!"
Russell:	You feel that way about Anita and about God.
Stephen:	That's right.
Russell:	That makes 1,000 percent sense. . . . So go with me here if you can. . . . When God hears that, when God hears that you're doing all this for God, and it feels like God's not doing anything back, when God feels you feeling that, how does God respond?
Stephen:	Nothing. I get nothing.
Russell:	So when you get nothing from God, nothing back, no response, what happens then?

Stephen:	It's a mix of things. Partly nothing. Just flat. Who cares? And partly mad.
Russell:	Can you go with that "mad" just a little bit? *["Mad" is an energy. It has potential to "do something." So I choose to focus here rather than on the inertia.]* Just give that some space. Let it build or expand some if it seems to be going in that direction. [Silence] And let me know what you notice.
Stephen:	I'm feeling mad at God.
Russell:	So just stay with that, and see if any words come from it.
Stephen:	"I'm mad. I'm just mad. And hurt. Why won't you help me? All I do, all I give, why won't you help me?" [He begins soft-pounding the sofa with his right fist.]
Russell:	So stay with that as long as it feels right. And maybe let your hand move as much or as strong as it wants to. Let it say whatever it wants to say to God too.
Stephen:	[His eyes are closed, his face in distress. He begins shaking his fist.]
Russell:	That's right. Whatever feels right, just keep saying it or doing it. [*It seems to me that Stephen has shifted from a left-brain state of consciousness to one that is more right-brain, meditative, and mindful.*]
Stephen:	[He keeps shaking his fist. Eventually this slows down, and his hand opens.]
Russell:	What's happening now?
Stephen:	I feel exhausted, but in sort of a good way.
Russell:	So just sense in to the exhaustion. It's OK to be tired. It makes sense that you're exhausted. Just feel it.

Stephen:	[He sighs loudly, several times, blowing his breath out and moaning softly. His eyes are still closed.]
Russell:	Is God still around?
Stephen:	Uh-huh.
Russell:	And what's God doing?
Stephen:	Just a little nearer.
Russell:	And when you feel God a little nearer, is there anything you want to say to God, or do?
Stephen:	"Help me trust you more." *[Asking for help is an act of agency. Success!]*
Russell:	You're asking God to help you trust God more.
Stephen:	Uh-huh.
Russell:	And what does God do in response?
Stephen:	Just stays a little nearer.
Russell:	Let's just let that happen, you feeling a little nearer to God. Asking God to help you trust. Take as much time with that as feels right.
Stephen:	[Silence now, softer breathing. He fidgets on the sofa and sits taller.] *[I consider the sitting taller a sign of increased active mode, of agency increasing and expressing itself somatically. I then try deepening that experience of agency by adding words to the somatic experience.]*
Russell:	And maybe go back to that prayer, "Help me trust you more," and add another: "If you do help me trust you more, how might you do that? How might I recognize your help?"
Stephen:	[Silence] God's not saying anything, but I do feel a sense of peace, and I'm also thinking that I've got to step out of the boat a little more. *[This is a reference to a story from the New Testament, where*

Jesus's disciple Peter steps out of a boat and walks on water to Jesus,[4] a sign of active faith.]

Stephen: I've got to take a few more chances, do some things I'm not comfortable doing.

Russell: Got it. So just let God know this is what you're thinking and see how God responds.

Stephen: [Silence] I still have that sense of peace.

A few minutes later, after Stephen returned to a more left-brain state of consciousness, I asked him what "doing something he's not comfortable doing" might mean in relation to Anita. He said he had not been visiting his son and grandson as much as he wanted, because she wanted Stephen with her, not elsewhere, and he wanted to change that pattern. I also asked him if there was anything uncomfortable he wanted to try in relation to God, and he said he wanted to sit a few minutes each day, just imagining God being with him.

Stephen eventually ended the relationship with Anita, but not quickly. It took another year, with lots of drama, many gains, and many retreats, before he stopped seeing her. Over that year, his confidence that his voice matters—with others, with himself, and with God—grew very slowly. The session described above was one of many in which I intervened to call forward and strengthen the active side of his personality.

THE WISDOM OF YOUR TRADITION

The two examples I've offered so far both involve me turning inward and finding a spiritual perspective that helped orient and guide me at particular clinical moments. But what happens when we turn inside and find . . . nothing? What about those times when, spiritually speaking, we find ourselves at a loss? Maybe we're in a not-so-great season of our own lives, or maybe the client is challenging us in a way that disorients or overwhelms us.

Here, I would suggest, is where it helps to be connected with the wisdom and practices of a spiritual tradition. All the world's great religions have provided meaning, comfort, and perspective to people for centuries, and they can be a resource for us when we listen for something inside of us and come up empty.

One of my favorite illustrations of this happened in a group supervision session I was leading. It's a wonderful example of people mining the gifts of their different religious traditions to offer help to a therapist who was feeling overwhelmed by her client's struggle to make sense of suffering.

The supervisee, Mary, is a Christian. She is twenty-eight years old and in her second year of practice. She has an engaging personality, is genuinely caring and highly conscientious, and works hard to help. Her clients sense all this in her, and the relationships she develops with them are exceptionally strong.

Mary's client is a fifty-one-year-old woman, Janet, who wants help with depression and with a spiritual struggle. Janet was abused as a child. She married and lost her first husband to cancer in her twenties. She had a serious car accident in her thirties, and she lives with chronic back pain as a result of that accident. Alongside this physical pain, and surely related to it, she has also been depressed for much of the past twenty years.

Janet has worked in retail and as an administrative assistant, but she is currently unemployed because her pain makes work unbearable. She takes medication for depression but nothing for pain. She remarried five years ago, a man she met at church, and this marriage is also a source of stress for her: her husband is critical of her for feeling bad as often as she does.

Janet attends a Baptist church, and her personal faith and faith community are both important to her. She speaks often in therapy about her spiritual questions: Why does God allow her to suffer so much? Why is she still having to endure such physical and emotional pain? What lessons might God be trying to teach her through all the hardship she has experienced?

Mary brought her work with Janet to group supervision and asked the group, "How can I help Janet make sense of her suffering when I don't understand it myself? I don't have the answers she is looking for, and I'm not sure how to help her find them."

Struggles with suffering, as we discussed in chapter 8, are often on our clients' minds, and it is always good when they feel free to voice these struggles in therapy. But Mary is right: the questions posed by suffering—where is God in this? why has God allowed it? what's required of me as a therapist in the midst of this?—have no easy answers, and we therapists can feel overwhelmed and overmatched by them.

Spiritual traditions have been grappling with these questions for centuries, of course, and they can be a resource for us as therapists. So I asked Mary and the group, "How does your spiritual tradition respond to suffering? When you encounter suffering, what does your tradition have to offer? What do people in your tradition say, and what do they do, in the presence of suffering? What wisdom would people in your tradition offer to Janet?"

Different group members responded:

"Casseroles. [The group laughed.] Seriously, we take food."

"We'd just be there for her. We might not have answers, but we'd stay connected and just be a presence with her."

"My faith says, 'Pray. Pray with her. Pray for her. Encourage her to pray.'"

"Mine says, 'Remember stories from the Bible where God was faithful, and stories of other people who have been brought through hard times. Tell those stories of deliverance.'"

"I think about the psalms, especially the psalms of lament. 'How long, O Lord?' 'Why is this happening to me, God?' 'Why have your forsaken me, God?' So my tradition, and all of them that claim the psalms, has this resource that says, 'You deal with suffering by telling God it's hard and you don't understand.'"

"My community doesn't say this directly, but it has a strong emphasis on service, on doing for others. I don't think anybody in my church would tell Janet, 'Oh, forget your own pain and needs, ignore those hard questions, just do something good for somebody else and you'll feel better.' Nobody would be that insensitive. But there is this unspoken wisdom that our own burdens get lighter when we give ourselves to the burdens of others."

I took notes on what they said and then summarized them. So the group says, "The wisdom of the ages about how to be with people who suffer is this":

"Bring food. Be caring and kind in a very practical way.

"Be present. You don't have to have answers, just be present.

"Pray. Turn your heart toward God.

"Remember the stories of deliverance. Remember times in your own life when it felt like God was with you, or God saw you through.

"Lament. It's important, it's good, it's sacred to tell God you're hurting and confused.

"Remember the world around you, and look for ways to care for others."

I then turned back to Mary.

Russell:	I'm wondering, from all that, what resonates with you and feels consistent with your spiritual tradition?
Mary:	All of it. What I learned as a child . . . and what my church says and does now . . . that's how my faith approaches these questions.
Russell:	So you're the therapist, and you're not gonna just give Janet a download of all these ideas, right? But how might you draw upon what your tradition teaches about suffering and how to be with people who suffer, to help you be with Janet and respond when she asks these hard questions?
Mary:	Well, I'm not gonna bring her food [the group laughs again], but I will continue to be kind to her. And this helps me see that kindness is a response to suffering. A legitimate response. It's something a group of wise people has decided is good thing to do.
Russell:	Yes.
Mary:	And when she asks these hard questions, I can just validate that they're good questions and that it's good for her to be thinking them and saying them aloud. She's a Christian, she knows the psalms. So I can tell her, "Hey, the Bible says it's OK to say these things." And I can ask her if there are

passages of Scripture that mean something to her and seem to help her with any of this.

Russell: That sounds good. What else?

Mary: I'm not gonna tell her she ought to do more for others, that if she'd do that she might not feel as focused on her pain. That would be cruel and stupid to say. But she does do things for other people all the time, and when she tells me about those things, I can just make more over it, get her to tell me more about it, how it affected her, things like that. And in general, just being with her. We say this all the time, don't we? Presence matters. The relationship heals. But this helps me see that that is something a spiritual community has decided is important too, not just therapy people.

Russell: So back to the question you brought: "How can I help her make sense of her suffering when I don't understand it myself? I don't have the answers she is looking for." How do you come at those questions now?

Mary: I don't have the answers she's looking for, but my tradition does. Her tradition does. All traditions do. And they're not A-B-C, 1-2-3 answers. They're answers you kind of have to live.

Russell: Right on.

Let me say two more things about this example. First, I want to reiterate what my intervention was with Mary: asking her, with the group's help, to consider how her religious tradition could be a resource for her. She was feeling short of spiritual resources herself, but we are never just on our own. There is always some community of wisdom around us to which we can turn for support, and I hope you'll draw upon yours as you do your work.

Second, I want to voice a personal opinion about suffering and the anguished questions we ask about it. I read the same Bible Mary reads, the same Bible Janet reads. And the question Mary and Janet are asking—"Why is this happening?"—I don't think the Bible ever answers it. The Bible has things to say about it. It tells stories about people who live through the worst losses and traumas you can imagine. Here and there it waxes poetically about it. But it never comes right out and says, clearly and unequivocally, "Here's how it all works. Here's why." In other words: the Bible doesn't have an easy answer for the question of suffering, and it's OK that we don't either. It's more than OK. Not having an answer is actually more biblical.

CONCLUSION

We've been talking about how to use our personal spiritual perspectives and the perspectives of our religious tradition to inform our work as therapists. We don't foist these perspectives upon our clients, but they are there all the same, behind the scenes, and they can help us tremendously in the work we do. I've shared three illustrations with you—two of times when I think my spirituality helped me offer better care to a client, a third of a time I think it helped a supervisee do so.

And now I want to invite you into some reflection of your own.

- What are some of your core spiritual beliefs, values, and practices?
- How do any of these inform a spiritual psychology: the way you understand people, the troubles they have, and what might help them?
- How do they affect how you do what you do as a therapist?

- Can you think of a time when your spiritual perspective affected what you said or did with a client?
- How much was that perspective operating behind the scenes? And how much was it declared in an upfront way?
- If there's a client you're struggling with currently, how might your spiritual perspective help you understand what's happening?

In the next chapter we'll turn these questions on their head a bit—less of how your spirituality affects your work with clients and more of how your clients' spirituality affects you. But before we go there, stay here awhile. Sit with the six questions above and see what happens.

12

Spiritual
Countertransference

IN THIS THIRD PART OF THE BOOK, WE'VE BEEN WORKING WITH the reality that our clients aren't the only ones in the room with a spiritual history, spiritual resources, and spiritual struggles. Nor are they the only ones whose spirituality might be causing harm in some way, to themselves or to others. All this is true of us, too, and that's why it's important, in any consideration of spiritually integrated psychotherapy, to give attention to the spirituality of the therapist.

In the previous two chapters we've focused on the spiritual perspectives that we therapists are conscious of—our beliefs, values, and practices—and how these influence our overall approach to therapy and our particular approach with particular clients.

In this chapter we'll focus on the perspectives that we're mostly *not* conscious of, not until they spontaneously and idiosyncratically make themselves known in some unique moment with a client. These are the involuntary, relationally rooted, sometimes-useful-sometimes-detrimental arisings of emotion, images, and physical sensations that the field of psychotherapy calls *countertransference*. In this chapter we'll talk about the spiritual dimension of countertransference, what we'll call *spiritual countertransference*.

WHAT IT IS

The name itself, "spiritual countertransference," may be new to you. But intuitively, you probably already know what it means.

One of your clients says something positive about a spiritual figure you admire. You feel a softening in your belly, notice that you really like this client, and see a quick flash in your mind of a place in the woods where you feel safe and happy.

Another says something positive about a spiritual figure you distrust. You feel yourself pulling back from this client a little, notice that you're holding your breath, and remember a teacher you had who was a bully.

Another client has been talking with you for weeks about a spiritual struggle, and she seems to be bogging down rather than moving through it. You feel anxious that maybe you're not doing enough to help, and you feel an urge to share with her some of the spiritual perspective that's helped you with this struggle.

Another is ultrareligious. Every other word—it's "the Lord" this, "the Lord" that. You want to get through to the real person behind all the religious talk, but you can't get anywhere close. It's about to drive you crazy.

Yet another made a difficult decision to leave a high-paying and ego-inflating job because he could feel it damaging his spirit. Now he's giving more time to his spiritual life, and he's flourishing. You feel inspired by the choice he made, the way he's living, and the radiance you feel in him.

Spiritual countertransference is all the responses you have to your clients' spirituality.[1] Your feelings (sad, mad, afraid, joyful, peaceful, attracted, bored, etc.), physical sensations, reasonable thoughts, bizarre thoughts, flashes of memory, sparks of intuition, music that begins playing in your head, voluntary and involuntary movement or impulses to move, spiritual awareness—all of that and more is spiritual countertransference.

And remember that the thing you're responding to—"your clients' spirituality"—can be explicitly or implicitly spiritual. A client rants against religion, or tells you he thinks his daughter is possessed by a demon, or denounces the "wishy-washy" religious people who have an anything-goes attitude about religious belief—all this is *explicit* spiritual material, and the response you have to that is spiritual countertransference. But say a client tells you her life is meaningless, or the story of delivering her first child, or her experience of being with her father as he died—this is *implicit* spiritual material, and your response to that is also spiritual countertransference.[2]

A HELP OR A HINDRANCE?

The actual term "spiritual countertransference" (or "religious countertransference") is rarely used in the psychotherapy literature, and when it is,[3] it's almost always described as an obstacle therapists must overcome. James Griffith's definition is representative: "Religious countertransference is an emotional response by a clinician toward a patient's religious language, beliefs, practices, rituals, or community that can diminish the effectiveness of treatment."[4]

And it is true, definitely, that spiritual countertransference can have a negative impact on our work. It can keep us from connecting with our client or understanding our client. It can make us tighten into a smaller version of ourselves and act out in some way: criticizing our client, withdrawing from our client, or playing God and overfunctioning on our client's behalf.

But spiritual countertransference can also make a positive contribution to our work. It can help us connect more deeply with our clients, attune more fully to their suffering, discern the presence and power of their resources, and fathom the emptiness of what they feel is missing. It is a way deep calls to deep,[5] and it is a wellspring of intuition from which our most creative interventions often flow. We do our best work—and are most nourished ourselves by our work—when our heart is open. Spiritual countertransference is part of how that happens.[6]

Whether our spiritual countertransference becomes a help or a hindrance depends on how we learn to work with it. And since each of us experiences spiritual countertransference in our own unique ways, each of us needs our own array of strategies to help us do that well.

STRATEGIES

Internally, there is no such thing as a wrong spiritual countertransference. The responses we have are the responses we have, and we should not judge them.

Externally, though—behaviorally, verbally, and nonverbally—we can definitely make some therapeutic mistakes. We can act out our spiritual countertransference in ways that harm our clients, harm us, and harm the work of therapy. We can push our spiritual perspective on a client. We can ignore a client's spirituality because we're uneasy with it. We can endorse a client's spirituality because it's similar to our own, but not be mindful of its drawbacks or shadow. And much, much more.

In this section, I want to name some strategies that might help you manage your never-wrong spiritual countertransference in ways that keep the therapy space safe and productive.

Cultivate Awareness

Spiritual countertransference becomes a problem only when we forget about it, so the foundational strategy for managing it is awareness. First, we need to be aware that important and meaningful responses are happening inside us at all times. Second, we need to know the different ways these important and meaningful responses make themselves known: through our thoughts, emotions, and bodies. In general, I try to give clients about 60 percent of my attention. The other 40 percent, I reserve for tracking my own experience. Countertransference matters that much, and it's important to stay awake to it—to its gifts and entanglements—as much as possible.[7]

Let's do a little awareness practice. Use 60 percent of your attention to read these next two clinical illustrations—the first is explicitly spiritual, the second implicitly spiritual—and 40 percent of your attention to notice what happens in you as you read.

Daniela grew up Roman Catholic, lost her younger brother to cancer when she was sixteen, got mad at God, left the church, began drinking heavily in her twenties, and got into AA in her mid-thirties. She's now in her fifties, has twenty years of sobriety, and came to you for help with moderate anxiety and mild depression. She told you she's been longing for a church but can't seem to find one. She likes AA and still goes, but she wants a *religious* community, not just a spiritual one.

In today's session she tells you that, for the past year, she's been having serendipitous run-ins with a local Baptist pastor. She's had a favorable impression of him and has been thinking about trying out his church. Last Saturday she and her husband were at Walmart and ran into him there. That sealed the deal for her. The next day, she and her husband visited the church and loved it. She tells you she can now see, in hindsight, how God was working little by little to help her find the church home she's been longing for.

What do you notice in yourself? Are you happy for her? Worried for her? Something else? Maybe even jealous? What's happening for you physically? Do you have a spiritual home? Are you aware of any spiritual longings of your own? What do you think about the idea that God was involved in helping all this come to be for her?

Here's a second example. In this one the spiritual issues are implicit rather than explicit. But take the 60/40 approach as you read this story of spiritual struggle and notice what happens.

Drew was sexually abused as a child by his older brother, began drinking and using drugs in his early teens, was addicted in his late teens, spent two years in prison in his twenties for burglary (to support his drug habit), began attending AA in prison, has been sober for ten years, and met his wife at AA in his early thirties. They have a two-year-old daughter together. He runs his own landscaping company; his wife is an accountant. They work hard and have bought a small house.

The shape his addictive behavior has taken in recent years involves looking at pictures of seductively clothed and posed preteen girls on the Internet. (When he was a preteen, his brother forced him to have sex with a preteen girl, while the brother watched.) His wife knows about his addiction/ obsession with young girls, and she worries that he will be an unsafe father to their daughter when she becomes older. He talks about this struggle with his AA sponsor, has attended some Sex Addicts Anonymous meetings as well, and manages months-long stretches where he does not engage in this behavior. When he breaks down and does look at pictures on his phone, he becomes highly enraged with himself. He punches himself, beats his head against a wall, and scratches at his skin. This behavior scares his wife.

In today's session he tells you about a relapse. He is so angry at himself, so down on himself, so hopeless of ever changing, that he thinks it's best if he leaves and cuts off all contact with his wife and daughter. This way his daughter won't be exposed to a dad like him and his wife won't have to feel the fear she feels.

What do you notice now? What is happening in your body? And what's it saying to you? What are you feeling? Fear? Judgment? Compassion? Admiration? Despair? Hope? Anger? And toward whom or what are you angry? Do you notice yourself moving toward Drew? Or pulling back? If you notice some of both, what's that like for you? Does he remind you of one your own clients? Or a family member or friend? What do you believe about basic human goodness or the flaws in human nature? What do you believe about people's ability to change?

Know Your Own Story

We also need to be aware of the kinds of spiritual countertransference responses that are typical for us. We don't have to keep getting ambushed, again and again, by the same responses. With some of them, we can be ready. Here it's helpful to reflect regularly on your spiritual history, your spiritual personality, your spiritual values, and your spiritual likes and dislikes—and consider how all these might affect your perception, the meanings you attribute, and the clinical decisions you make.

Here's a personal example. I grew up Southern Baptist in the 1960s and '70s. My parents took my brothers and me to church three times a week—Sunday morning, Sunday night, and Wednesday night. I sang hymns. (More than anything else, I think Christian faith got sung into me.) I learned the Bible, a good bit of it by heart. I watched people take care of each other and do good things for people they did not know. I also heard sermons about hell, noticed the absolute whiteness of the churches we attended, and heard my seventh-grade Sunday school teacher warn my friends and me about a "faggot" in the church who was preying on boys our age.

At home, my parents expressed their devotion to the faith, but they were more open-minded than the Southern Baptist party line. When I asked if they thought people who weren't Christians would go to hell, they said no, they didn't think God would do that. They were troubled by the racial segregation of our church—my parents were both public school educators in a majority-black South Carolina school system—and they supported me the few times I brought black friends to church. All in all, they considered it a good thing to be part of church and take me with them, but neither of them was a hook-line-and-sinker person.

What my parents' example modeled for me—and through them, what also got sewn into my bones—is that it's possible to take what's positive from a religious tradition but not be captive to the parts that aren't so positive. Because of their example, I think, it's usually not hard for me to listen to all sorts of religious ideas, hear the good in them (or the deep human need expressed in them) and not be terribly triggered. (Another reason that's usually easy for me, of course, is that I was, and am, white, male, upper-middle-class, straight, and a member of a spiritual majority—all factors of privilege that make me feel less vulnerable in the world and mean I have less cause to be sensitive or defensive.)

The way this is relevant for me, countertransferentially, and the reason I'm telling you, is that my "even harmful religion doesn't necessarily have to harm you" experience can make me less aware of and less empathic with the experience of clients (and supervisees and friends) who have experienced spiritual injury or who are triggered by some noxious spiritual ideology or practice. When I hear another person getting reactive, offended, or angry about something spiritual, something in me thinks, *Well, just don't let that bother you. Don't waste your energy. You be you and keep moving.* This is not—spoiler alert—usually a helpful response. And knowing about this blind spot in my own spiritual history has helped me slow down and feel empathy for clients who are agitated about someone else's beliefs or values, and prevented more than one therapeutic rupture.[8]

So, if you've got a few minutes right now, take a moment and do some reflecting about your own spiritual experience. Grab a sheet of paper and make some notes in response to these prompts. Don't edit; just jot down whatever comes readily to mind.

- Five things about some place you lived as a child
- Five things about your spiritual home
- One of your spiritual mentors
- One of your best spiritual memories
- One of your hardest spiritual memories
- Two or three words that describe your spiritual personality (trusting/skeptical, homebody/explorer, cognitive/emotional, reliant on external authority/trusting your inner knowing, active/contemplative, drawn to groups/drawn to solitude, etc.)
- Two things you currently believe, spiritually
- One thing you currently struggle with, spiritually
- Someone who's frightened or hurt you spiritually

Relatedly, it's also helpful to know the kinds of spirituality or religion that tend to trigger us. Here is a list of some of common spiritual triggers. Some I know from personal experience, others from the reports of supervisees and colleagues. Take another minute and notice which clients are the most activating for you—the client

- Who is disparaging of or disinterested in spirituality
- Whose every other word is spiritual
- Who is deeply religious and is in a season of doubt—a dark night of the soul
- Who is in a spiritual high place (and maybe you're not)
- Who is angry with God and speaks it freely

- Who is angry with God but can't admit it
- Who feels hopeless
- Who is openly gay[9]
- Who is gay but fighting against it for religious reasons
- Who wants you to be a spiritual authority for him and answer his spiritual questions
- Who considers herself your spiritual superior, who tolerates you but believes she is spiritually more advanced than you are
- Who is spiritual in a way you used to be

And here's one last question: Which of those prompts evokes the most charge for you? Perhaps a good charge, evoking connection with something positive in your spirituality? A bad charge, evoking connection with something negative or painful? Or an absence of charge: blankness or confusion (which are perhaps the most important charges of all to notice)?

Awareness of our typical and atypical spiritual countertransference is the foundation. We can't manage what's happening without noticing what's happening. But after awareness, then what?

Befriend Within

Whatever we become aware of in ourselves—our thoughts, feelings, and physical sensations—a pretty good next step is to befriend it. Acknowledge it, accept it, relate to it, and try to understand it—just as you would with a friend.

Turn toward your reaction, and ask it, as you would a friend, if it can help you understand it a little more. Maybe ask how it has come to feel the way it does, or how come it's showing up right now, at just this moment, with this client.

Maybe it's there to protect you. What your client is saying, the way he's saying it, or the way he's acting may remind you of someone who's hurt you or frightened you before.

Maybe your reaction is serving your ego in some way. Perhaps you're comparing yourself in some way to this client, favorably or unfavorably. And your reaction—admiring the client, judging the client, feeling envy or shame in relation to the client—might be connected to one of the self-evaluating or self-serving projects of ego.

Whatever you learn, the important thing is to be curious: ask, listen, and understand yourself without judgment. Then maybe ask this response you're having what it needs: what needs to happen so that your countertransference dials back a little and allows you to return to a state of openheartedness? Perhaps it wants assurance from you that you're paying attention to boundaries. Perhaps the client's need has helped awaken you to a need in yourself, and your countertransference is asking that you give more care to it. Perhaps it has wisdom to offer that will help you help your client and just wants you to listen to it for a moment. Maybe it wants support from one of your spiritual resources. Whatever this part of you might be wanting, and speaking up to ask for, see if you can help that to happen.

Here's another personal example. Sometimes I feel judgmental and impatient with clients whose spiritual personality (and overall personality) is fairly cognitive. These are the clients who come at spirituality more philosophically than experientially. For the most part, I am fairly empathic with these clients. I appreciate the sense of safety and all the good information their heads provide them, and I am fairly gentle and patient in the way I relate to them. But once in a while, I'll find myself restless and irritated with clients who aren't getting anywhere because they're stuck in their head.

As I've noticed this tendency, I've learned to befriend my frustration and impatience. Here's what I've come to understand.

I am, at heart, a heart person. (Maybe we all are, originally.) But at the age of six, I got kidnapped and brainwashed by an educational system that privileges head over heart. I adapted

to this circumstance, quite thoroughly and somewhat success-
fully, and I lost much of my native connection with heart, body,
and spirit. Even my spiritual education was head-focused. In
college and at seminary, I was taught to read the Bible critically
and skeptically, and I relied on this academic approach to spirituality to guide me for the first fifteen years I was a minister.
Poor me! And poor the people I cared for!

Eventually, though, by the grace of God, the patience of
friends and family, and the necessities of this crazy profession
I ended up in, I reconnected with my heart. I'm glad I know all
I know intellectually, but I feel some regret and ache about the
years I lived without connection to inner spiritual knowing.
I also feel, sometimes, a bit of resentment toward academic,
head-based spirituality (and academic, head-based anything),
and I now prefer experiential approaches to everything—spirituality, psychotherapy, and book-writing included.

So now, when I'm with head-people, and I notice the heart-
part of me feeling irritated and impatient, I try to befriend that
heart-part of myself. I let it know I understand how exiled and
undernourished it felt for so many years. I validate that it worries
I might get sucked back into that imbalanced world, or that it
wants to change the head-person I'm with as quickly as possible.
I let my heart know I appreciate its worry, but that its place in me
is secure, that I can stay connected with it even in the presence
of all this head energy that used to dominate me and repress my
heart energy. ("See?" I say to my heart. "We're connected right
now.") And then—on my better days, anyway—by befriending my own feelings, I'm able to stay connected with my clients
and work with them at the pace and in the manner they require,
which is the only pace and manner that actually works.

Seek Support (Be Friended)

As helpful as it is to befriend our countertransference responses
internally, and as necessary as it is to do that in the middle of

a session when it's just you and your client, it's also essential to seek the support of colleagues, friends, a supervisor, or a therapist. When you notice that you're dreading seeing a certain client, or feeling shame in the presence of a certain client, or feeling superidentified and invested in a moral choice a client is facing, or having any sort of response to your client's spirituality that you can feel is in the way, it's always a good idea to talk this through with someone you trust.

Early in my work as a therapist, I would feel nervous when I worked with extremely religious clients. I was nervous they would ask me what I believed and that whatever I said in response—whether I told them plainly or whether I deflected and asked what that question meant to them—they would find it lacking. For a while, I understood my nervousness in an economic sense. I was building a practice, and my family needed the money those clients were paying me. I didn't want to lose them!

But I told some friends and a supervisor about my nervousness, and as I explored it with them, I came to understand that I was not at peace with my own spiritual evolution. The Christian faith that had been sung into my bones was still there, but not in the same way it was when I was younger. It wasn't *just* Christian anymore. There was some Buddhism, Hinduism, Taoism, Judaism, Sufism, and more also in the mix. Talking about my nervousness with these trusted others helped me understand that I was uneasy with my own spiritual journey: was it OK that I had become interspiritual in the way I had, drinking from the wells of many traditions? I was projecting this uneasiness onto my clients, imagining that they would judge me and find me spiritually unsuitable to do the work they needed. I didn't automatically make complete peace with the spiritual path my life had taken, but I did stop worrying about whether my clients were thinking I was a spiritual apostate. And as that anxiety eased, I found it so much easier to connect with them in a meaningful, spiritual way.

Educate Yourself

I'll be short and sweet on this point. The more we know about spiritualities other than our own, the less threatening they will become and the less reactive we will be to them. It's natural to feel guarded in the presence of differentness. But the more we learn about the other, the less other that person becomes. If you want to work with clients of diverse spiritual perspectives— and if you're in a rural area where you might be one of the only mental health options available, it might be necessary that you do so, whether you want to or not—you need to get to know diverse spiritual perspectives.[10]

Read as much as you can. Huston Smith's *The World's Religions* is now over fifty years old, but it has been updated over time, and it's still hard to beat as a one-source volume for learning about the major religious traditions. There are excellent video resources available through the PBS website and on YouTube. But there's truly no substitute for firsthand experience: visiting a church, synagogue, mosque, or sangha you know little about; introducing yourself to their leaders; and asking for introductions to people who might help you learn more about their religion.

Tend to Ruptures

Sooner or later, despite your best efforts to manage your countertransference, you're going to act out and create a therapeutic rupture.

It might be a small rupture. Sometimes, for instance, I'll feel excited that a client is "growing" spiritually. But in my excitement, I forget that she might also be grieving the spiritual home she's leaving. For a little while, I get ahead of her and don't notice the signs of her grief.

Or it might be a large rupture. I once had a client get very aggressive with me, complaining that I was not being clear with his wife that her faith required her to stay in their marriage. He referenced the biblical story where King David orders his soldier Uriah to the front line of battle, where Uriah was killed, so that David could marry Uriah's wife, Bathsheba. The client said that I was David, he was Uriah, and his wife was Bathsheba. She was the only thing he had, like Bathsheba was all Uriah had, and I was trying to take her away from him. I knew a rupture might be happening the moment I noticed that the index finger on my right hand was making stabbing motions at him while I challenged his analogy.

That was a rupture beyond repair, but most ruptures are small enough that, if we notice them, we can mend them. The onus is on us to acknowledge what's happened and, if we think it'll be useful, to apologize or describe from our perspective what happened. Here's an example.

Anna is depressed. Her depression has more than one cause, as is often the case, but one of the large contributors is her recent loss of faith. I won't relate the details of how she lost her faith, but she feels both a massive hole in her life and a determination not to be taken in, ever again, by any spiritual charlatan. Wherever she ends up spiritually, it's important to her that she get there by way of her own inner knowing, not by the recommendation of any outside-herself authority.

In a recent session, she reached a point of great pain and began weeping. She closed her eyes, dropped her head, and sobbed. I sat with her in complete silence for two minutes, noticing her, noticing the sensation and energy in my body, giving special attention to the energy in my heart, which is for me a way of praying.

Then I began to get a little antsy, and I started thinking that maybe I ought to say something. Maybe the silent spiritual energy in the room wasn't enough. Maybe she needed to hear an actual human voice, even softly, to know she was not alone. I wasn't sure what to do, but I began saying softly, "Mmm."

Then: "Yes, stay with it, and let that happen." And eventually: "Notice if those tears are connected with any memory, or any longing, or any words."

Anna continued to weep, but within a minute she stopped and told me what she had been thinking as she cried.

I still felt uneasy, though. I wasn't sure if my speaking and offering a little direction had been helpful to her, or if it would have been better for me to have continued supporting her silently. Especially since one of her "heart of the matter" issues is whether she gets to have her own experience, or whether her experience will be directed by someone outside herself, I thought it was important that I acknowledge the way this issue was playing out between us. I told her about the uncertainty I had experienced and asked for her feedback. I asked specifically, "Did my voice enter the space too soon? Too late? Or at just the right time?"

She told me that the weeping she does with me is very, very helpful. She feels something healing in her as she does that. She also said that the question I had asked about her tears had been helpful, but that I had offered it a little too soon. It would have been better to have had a little more time for her emotion to crescendo, crest, and drop in an arc of its own.

I thanked her for being honest with me about that, affirmed that I want to help her but need her feedback to know how best to do that, and invited her to let me know when I need to make some adjustment even if I'm not aware enough to ask. She breathed deeply, and her face looked stronger to me.

Listen for Help

Spiritual countertransference isn't always an intrusion of our own issues into the therapy relationship. Sometimes it's the way empathy happens—a way we come to feel what our clients feel or know what they know. Sometimes it's the way intuition happens—a way we come to know something our clients are not yet able to let themselves know. And sometimes spiritual countertransference is the bearer of therapeutic inspiration.

It would be a shame to miss all the information and assistance our countertransference has to offer. So whenever emotion, physical sensation, thought, memory, or any of the other countertransference languages speak up in us, it's helpful to wonder what they might be telling us—about our clients, about what they need, about how we might relate to them in a therapeutic way. This is a step beyond befriending our countertransference. This is receiving its wisdom.

Lamar is chronically stressed. His outer world provides him plenty of cause: he works a high-demand job and cares for several family members with serious health problems. Recently, though, things have settled down considerably at work, and his sick family members are needing less from him. But he still feels stressed as ever, as if nothing around him had changed. As he told me this, he spoke quickly, like he usually does. His face remained on alert (his eyebrows high), and his body looked stiff and tense.

As he talked, what I noticed inside myself was a wide plain of stillness in my chest, spreading out inside me and beyond me. This was my countertransference to his implicit spiritual state of distress. I enjoyed it, savored it, and I understood it to be saying, "This is what he's missing. This is what he wants."

So I said to him, "What I'm hearing is that your outer world is slowing down, but your inner world is still running ninety miles per hour. You're not feeling any of the stillness in yourself."

"That's right," he said, "I'm not." He paused. "I wish I could slow down inside"—and here he extended his arms and made something of bowl with his hands, as if he were holding an invisible basketball—"but I can't."

When he made that gesture with his hands, a fragment of a song flashed through my brain: "He's got the whole world in his hands." I understood it to be saying, "This is how responsible he feels, like he's got to take care of the whole world."

I mirrored his gesture back to him and sang the first line of the song: "He's got the whole world in his hands." Then I added, "It's really hard."

"Wow," he said, and everything about him stopped a moment. He did the gesture again, then dropped his hands in his lap and looked at me. His eyes seemed to be reaching for me, which I interpreted as a request for help.

I then started hearing this line from the song: "He's got the itty-bitty baby in his hands." And I thought, *That's his help.*

So I said, "Do you want to try something and see if it might slow you down a little on the inside?"

"Sure."

"Right out there," I said, and held my hands in front of me in the way he had been. "Right there, where sometimes you feel like you're carrying the whole world, imagine a baby sleeping. A very small baby, perfectly still. And just watch it. Watch it with your eyes. Watch it with your heart. Very slowly. And try letting[11] yourself become as still as that little baby."

Then we were silent together for a minute. I still felt the great plain of stillness there in me. I was watching the baby too.

Then Lamar took a deep breath.

"A little slower, huh?"

"Yes." He took another deep breath. "A little stiller."

"So don't do anything. Just let yourself enjoy this."

My countertransference is not always so wonderfully attuned, of course. In fact, it's usually not, and there are regular ruptures I need to repair. But sometimes we just have a sense that what we're experiencing can be of some use to our client. So if we're willing to carry it lightly, offer it experimentally, notice whether it deepens the client's exploration or interrupts it, and adjust accordingly, our spiritual countertransference can be a wellspring of wisdom. Not to mention—a cause for gratitude and wonder.

CONCLUSION

Psychotherapy is an interaction between humans, not between robots or protocols, and it is the motley and marvelous humanness of both persons, spirituality included, that makes therapy both possible and complicated.

It is our limbically resonant human nervous system that makes connection between two people possible. And that same limbically resonant human nervous system—with its complex associative-memory network, wherein hundreds and thousands of associations, each of them brimming with cognition, emotion, and physical sensation, can be evoked by a single word, a tilt of the head, or a slant of light—makes connection complicated.

All the gifts and complications of human connection show up in the therapy relationship, and I have shared a few thoughts about the spiritual dimension of your side of that relationship, what we call "spiritual countertransference." I have offered strategies for navigating its challenges, but I've also encouraged you to welcome it as a teacher and guide.

Like all the other chapters in this book, this one has just scratched the surface of a matter we could spend days and days discussing together, in long, searching, illuminating, humbling, and hilarious conversation. And at the end of those days, we would know, in the way we know about matters of deep mystery, that there is much more we don't know. But we would have been enlarged and enriched and amazed by the conversation, and the topic, and the company. And I hope at least a little of that feels true after your time in this chapter.

13

Conclusion

"How do I do that?" How do I work with spirituality in psychotherapy? How do I recognize the ten thousand ways spirituality presents itself in a human life, increase its positive effects in my clients' lives, and lessen the harm it might be causing?

This is the question with which we began, and in the pages between that beginning and this ending, I've offered a framework in which you can live into answers that work for you and your practice.

The framework I've offered includes a bit of theory, lots of skills and strategies, and an ample portion of my own spiritual values and assumptions. I won't review every element of that framework in these final pages, but I'll highlight a few that are primary:

- **Being spiritual is a given, not a choice,** no more than being physical, psychological, or social are choices.
- **We can have a spiritual conversation with a client without either of us using an explicitly spiritual word.**

- As often as possible, which is almost always, **we work within our clients' spiritual frame of reference**, learning what's true, real, and meaningful for them and using the language they use.

- As often as possible, **we keep directing our clients back to experience**, nudging them, gently but firmly, from "known already" to "knowing now," to the liminal space where cognition meets emotion and physical experience. Working experientially and mindfully is a way to help our clients' spirituality be even more of a transforming resource in their lives.

- **Our own spirituality matters too**, and there are ways to draw upon it—for wisdom and for self-care—without imposing it on our clients.

- **We move always at the speed of trust.** Knowing what trust looks like when it's happening, what it looks like when it's not, and how to earn and deserve your clients' trust are foundational skills for working with spirituality.

- **Being smart and impressive is no match for being respectful, humble, and kind.** The most helpful question for working with spirituality in psychotherapy is also the simplest: "Would you tell me more about that?"

LAST WORDS

Whether you are a seasoned therapist or a relative beginner, I hope the framework I've offered here, and the way I've offered it, have helped you feel more confident to do this work in the way that only you can do it. In that hope, I want to use these last moments with you to say three more things.

First, don't stop here. This book is but a beginning. Go get yourself more support. Read some of the wonderful books about psychotherapy and spirituality I've referenced throughout this book—and find some others I've not, and tell me about them. Keep your eyes open for workshops, conferences, or extended trainings.[1] Find a supervisor or consultant you trust to talk with about your cases. Call together some colleagues, read something together, or discuss cases together, or practice together some of the skills from this book. There is so much more to learn, and it is so worth learning.

Second, consider letting your therapy practice be a spiritual practice. You may be familiar with the term "spiritual practice" and already see your work in this way. But perhaps it's new to you, so let me define it and describe what I mean.

A *spiritual practice* is anything we do with the intention of growing ourselves (or, allowing ourselves to be grown) spiritually. It might be something we set aside time to do—like meditating, attending worship somewhere, or performing some act of service. Or it might be an attitude or posture we weave into our everyday activities—walking with mindfulness, practicing gratitude, praying for strangers, softening our anger when it arises, or attuning our hearts to see in other people the face of God.

Treating our therapy practice as a spiritual practice means coming to the therapy hour as a time not just for our clients to grow and change but for us to do that too. It's not just "them" who are having the opportunity to soften their constriction, compulsion, fear, hardness of heart, hopelessness, and desire to control everything. We are too.

I cannot tell you how many times I have had this experience. A client is ready to do a deep piece of work: ready consciously and with intention, or ready with no conscious intention, ready because some strong emotion in them, with a mind of its own, senses an opportunity to be held, heard, and healed. But I'm not ready. Maybe I'm tired. Maybe my last hour was difficult and I feel fragile or rattled. Maybe I'm not sure I'll know what to do. Whatever the reason, I just don't feel confident I've got what it takes to be present to the intensity I know will be part of these next thirty or forty minutes. Will I make myself available anyway? Will I say yes to taking the next steps with this client?

Sometimes the answer is no, of course. Some days, I choose to play it safe. But sometimes the answer is yes. Even though I'm not sure it's going to go well or be OK, I say yes. And I find, again and again, that when I say yes to these moments, when I agree to proceed—not by my own sense of strength, confidence, or power, but proceed all the same—without fail, *without fail,* I am given the ability to do my part, something important happens for the client, and I am nourished by what unfolds.

In this way, the practice of therapy has strengthened my capacity to trust. It has also grown my ability to be patient when I feel lost, to keep trying when I feel helpless, to ask for help (from a client or a colleague) when I'm not sure what's going on or what to do next, to forgive my clients when they hurt me, and to be forgiven when I hurt them.

I'm encouraging you to receive this as one of the gifts of your job too. Let your practice be a practice.

Third, and last, I want to thank you for caring enough about your clients to read this book. Ours is a culture, it seems to me, that pulls people away from connection with inwardness, depth, and meaning. There are relentless pressures to do more, juggle more, produce more, acquire more, and protect more, and the gravitational pull of these various pressures is centrifugal, taking us further and further from center and from spiritual awareness. Even so, there remains a centripetal hunger, a desire for connection and meaning that deepens, unifies, integrates, and empowers. It is difficult to live with a hunger like this when we feel little hope of its satisfaction or little capacity for nourishing it. Many in our day, and probably in earlier days also, have given up on their spiritual longing. They dissociate from it and do not allow themselves to feel it or express it. But it is there all the same, consciously or unconsciously, and from time to time people do speak of it, or from it. This is an act of great vulnerability and courage—to feel the deep longing for spiritual connection and meaning, to breathe it aloud, to look into another's eyes and see if they feel it too. And when people risk in these ways—risk letting this spiritual hunger arise in themselves, or risk speaking of it to their therapist—it is important that their risk be met with authentic, tender, humble, human companionship.

So thank you for wanting to do that, and wanting to do it well. I hope this book helps you meet your clients in those moments when their hunger for the sacred reveals itself. And I hope as well that the work you do is nourishment for the sacred hunger that is your own.

Acknowledgments

SO MANY GOOD PEOPLE HELPED BRING THIS BOOK TO BIRTH. Here are some of them:

The clients who've come to talk with me through the years. You have been my patient teachers.

The CareNet Residents and other supervisees who've trusted me to support your work. When it comes to spirituality and psychotherapy, you're the ones who've helped me separate the wheat from the chaff.

These friends and colleagues at CareNet Counseling and Wake Forest Baptist Health: Steve Scoggin, who hired me to develop the CareNet Residency and teach the material that eventually became this book; Bryan Hatcher and Gary Gunderson, my other bosses at CareNet and Wake, who have fully supported this project; and Emily Viverette, Rosalind Bradley, and Robert Willis, strong partners in teaching and nourishing a next generation of spiritually integrated psychotherapists.

These friends and colleagues who offered feedback on various chapters and drafts of this book: Nathan Blake, Aquita

Burrus, Carol Ebron, Jeremy Fox, Morgan Goforth, Amy Greene, Bill Harkins, Anita Harrison, Denise Merritt, Patricia Paronett-Ballard, Camila Pulgar, Shelley Ratterman, Larry Rosenberg, and Joe Wilkerson.

These friends and colleagues who were ridiculously generous with guidance and encouragement along the path to publication: Ken Pargament and Jill Snodgrass. I can't pay you back, but I'll pay it forward.

My friends, colleagues, and mentors in these communities of learning and service: the American Association of Pastoral Counselors; ACPE: The Standard for Spiritual Care and Education; the Internal Family Systems community; the Sensorimotor Psychotherapy community; the Solihten Institute; the Partnership for Pastoral Counseling; and Circle of Mercy congregation.

The terrific team at Templeton Press: Susan Arellano, Angelina Horst, Trish Vergilio, and Dan Reilly. You made this book a much better book and, for that matter, a book at all.

My brother-in-law and running partner, Mark Siler. You talked me through many a stuck place on the trails at Warren Wilson. And Lady kept the bears away.

My wife, Jeanine Siler Jones: first reader, best reader, take-a-break advisor, partner of my heart. We have birthed each other.

And our children, Peyton and Walton. At least once a day, in some moment of decision or difficulty, I ask myself, "What would they do right now?"

Great, heart-felt, heart-full thanks to all of you.

And to the All in all.

Notes

Chapter 1

1. One of the most down-to-earth therapists of the twentieth century understood this. Donald Winnicott was a pediatrician and psychoanalyst in London in the 1930s through the 1970s. He once wrote, "You may cure your patient and not know what it is that makes him or her go on living. It is of first importance for us to acknowledge openly that absence of psychoneurotic illness may be health but it is not life" (Winnicott, "Location of Cultural Experience," 100). He also said, "We disagree with Freud. He was for 'curing symptoms.' We are concerned with whole living and loving persons" (quote attributed to Winnicott by Harry Guntrip; cited in Mendez and Fine, "Short History," 361).

2. Berry, "Peace of Wild Things," 69.

3. Marshall Mahan Siler Jr., 1962–2017.

Chapter 2

1. Pew Research Center, "America's Changing Religious Landscape."

2. Oliver, *New and Selected Poems*, 1:94.

Chapter 3

1. John Wesley (1703–1791), his brother Charles, and George Whitefield were the founders of Methodism.

2. Abraham Heschel (1907–1972) was a Jewish rabbi and theologian. I could not locate this quote, nor could the friend who quoted it to me. But the point is not to get the quote right. The point is the experience this person is describing.

3. At least one of the people who said this was a monk named Theophan. In *Into the Silent Land*, Martin Laird quotes Theophan as saying, "You must descend from your head to your heart," 27.

4. John 21:25.

Chapter 4

1. Pargament, *Spiritually Integrated Psychotherapy*, 32.

2. Orr, *Concerning the Book*, 29.

3. Additionally, on the human side of the relationship, while "the search for the sacred" acknowledges that people seek God, seek growth, seek meaning, and the like, it leaves out the way people also don't-seek, don't-search, and actively avoid these matters. In the same way that our understanding of psychology is large enough to include denial, dissociation, and other workings of the unconscious, our understanding of spirituality needs to be large enough to include people who ignore, avoid, or evade God, as well as people who don't orient toward the world in any conscious spiritual sense. "I'm not a spiritual person" is itself an expression of spirituality.

4. This is the way I first heard it. The source seems to be from a 1948 book called *Personality in Nature, Society, and Culture*, by Henry A. Murray and Clyde Kluckhohn. The original wording was in the accepted style of that time: "Like all other men, like some other men, like no other man."

5. Griffith, *Religion That Heals*, 20.

6. *Ruach* in Hebrew, *pneuma* in Greek. In the Bible, then, the Holy Spirit is also the Holy Breath and the Holy Wind.

7. Rohr, *Immortal Diamond*, 29.

8. Griffiths, *River of Compassion*, 7.

9. A version of this story frames David Foster Wallace's 2005 commencement speech at Kenyon College, "This Is Water." And here's a related quoted from Thomas Merton's rendering of the Taoist sage Chuang Tzu: "Fishes are born in water / Man is born in Tao" (*Way of Chuang Tzu*, 65).

10. 1 Samuel 3.

11. Matthew 26:40.

12. This is the question my friend's client asks in chapter 1.

Chapter 5

1. Porges and Howes, "Wearing Your Heart." Here's a quote from that interview: "Good therapy and good social relations, good parenting, good teaching, it's all about the same thing—how do you turn off defensiveness? When you turn defense systems off, you have accessibility to different cortical areas for more profound understanding, learning, and skill development."

2. If you believe that everything is spiritual, that there is a spiritual dimension embedded in all reality, then it follows that all language is implicitly spiritual. (The act of speaking itself—the impulse to make contact with others and convey something meaningful to them—is, in some understandings—mine included—a spiritual act.) But some not-explicitly-spiritual words have more spiritual resonance than others. They bring a fullness to our hearts or a lump in our throats in ways that others do not.

3. See Kahneman's work on priming in *Thinking*.

4. Griffith and Griffith, *Encountering the Sacred*, 46.

5. This question, and the three that follow, are from Pargament's *Spiritually Integrated Psychotherapy*, 210.

Chapter 6

1. Even the therapeutic relationship, which is the foundation for everything else that happens, is an intervention.

2. I've had many good teachers help me learn this balanced approach: clients, supervisees, supervisors, and some excellent written resources. These publications have helped me most: Griffith, *Religion That Heals*; Griffith and Griffith, *Encountering the Sacred*; Hodge, "Implicit Spiritual Assessment"; Pargament, *Spiritually Integrated Psychotherapy*; Plante, *Spiritual Practices in Psychotherapy*; Richards and Bergin, *Spiritual Strategy*; and Sperry, *Spirituality in Clinical Practice*. I'll occasionally reference one of these works here, but for the most part what I'm presenting you is a condensed and synthesized adaptation of these good resources, all of which I recommend to you as you have time to go deeper.

3. Plante, *Spiritual Practices in Psychotherapy*, 63–64, cites five instruments that he considers usable in clinical settings: the Brief Multidimensional Measure of Religiousness/Spirituality, the Santa Clara Strength of Religious Faith Questionnaire, the Duke University Religious Index, the Religious Commitment Inventory—10, and the RCOPE and Brief RCOPE.

4. Most of these questions come from Griffith and Griffith, *Encountering the Sacred*, 46; Hodge, "Implicit Spiritual Assessment," 227; and Pargament, *Spiritually Integrated Psychotherapy*, 218.

5. This is one of my favorite questions. I sometimes introduce it this way, "We're all different physically, and I believe we're all different spiritually. God connects with some of us through church, some of us through nature, some of us through reading, some of us through food, and on and on. What channels does God play on for you?" This introduction and question are often life-changing for people who've been taught that God must be approached in some prescribed way.

6. Most of these questions come from Pargament, *Spiritually Integrated Psychotherapy*, 225–26. See those pages for a complete list of explicit spiritual assessment questions.

7. Pargament, *Spiritually Integrated Psychotherapy*, p. 212.

8. Welwood, *Toward a Psychology of Awakening*, 11–15.

9. Griffith and Griffith, *Encountering the Sacred*, 88, 89.

Chapter 7

1. For example: to help them strengthen their capacity for emotional regulation, increase their experience of agency, deepen their sense of hope, or access basic resources like shelter, food, healthcare, or transportation.

2. Throughout this book, when I share my own thinking within clinical dialogue, I italicize my thoughts and place them in brackets. Nonverbal expressions appear in nonitalicized bracketed type.

3. Ogden and Fisher, *Sensorimotor Psychotherapy,* 137.

4. Kabat-Zinn, *Wherever You Go,* 4.

5. Some excellent books on mindfulness are Nhat Hanh, *Miracle of Mindfulness;* Kabat-Zinn, *Wherever You Go;* and Williams and Penman, *Mindfulness.*

6. Some excellent podcasts that include teachings on mindfulness are *Mindfulness Mode* by Bruce Langford; *10% Happier* with Dan Harris; and *Tara Brach* by Tara Brach.

7. You can find an MBSR class near you at https://www.umassmed.edu/cfm/mindfulness-based-programs/mbsr-courses/find-an-mbsr-program/.

8. See Goleman and Davidson, *Altered Traits,* for a great summary of the current state of research on the benefits of meditation. They note that while scientific research strongly suggests the benefits I have cited, most of the promising scientific studies still need to be replicated and tested on larger sample sizes. Even so, while we await more rock-solid scientific proof, Goleman and Davidson remain strong advocates of meditation as a health-positive practice.

9. Three of the many good books on Christian meditation are Finley, *Christian Meditation;* Keating, *Invitation to Love;* and Bourgeault, *Heart of Centering Prayer.*

10. Three of the innumerable good books on Buddhist meditation are Kornfield, *Meditation for Beginners;* Chodron, *How to Meditate;* and Nhat Hanh, *Peace Is Every Step.*

11. Helminski, *Living Presence*; Bair, *Living from the Heart*.

12. These books all teach meditation without any religious framework: Harris, *Meditation for Fidgety Skeptics*; Reninger, *Meditation Now*; and Taft, *The Mindful Geek*. Additionally, clients and colleagues have recommended these smartphone apps to me: Headspace, Insight Timer, and Stop, Breathe & Think.

13. Richards and Bergin, *Spiritual Strategy*, 261.

14. Tanakh is an acronym of the first Hebrew letter of three traditional subdivisions: Torah ("Teaching," also known as the Five Books of Moses), Nevi'im ("Prophets") and Ketuvim ("Writings").

15. Gubi, *Prayer in Counselling and Psychotherapy*; Magaletta, "Prayer in Psychotherapy"; La Torre, "Prayer in Psychotherapy"; Rossiter-Thornton, "Prayer in Psychotherapy"; Richards and Bergin, *Spiritual Strategy*.

16. Gubi, *Prayer in Counselling*.

Chapter 8

1. Pargament, Presentation.

2. Abu-Raiya et al., "Prevalence."

3. Abu-Raiya et al., "Robust Links."

4. Abu-Raiya et al., "Examination."

5. Balboni and Balboni, *Hostility to Hospitality*, 28.

6. Desai and Pargament, "Predictors."

7. Pargament, *Spiritually Integrated Psychotherapy*, 112.

8. Ibid., 112–13.

9. Ibid., 113.

10. Matthew 27:46. Jesus is quoting Psalm 22:1.

11. Mother Teresa, *Come Be My Light*, 187.

12. Renzetti, "Bruce Springsteen."

13. See Ogden and Fisher, *Sensorimotor Psychotherapy*, 137.

14. I highly recommend a book by Benedictine nun Joan Chittister titled *Welcome to the Wisdom of the World and Its Meaning for You*. She pairs insight from Hinduism, Buddhism,

Judaism, Christianity, and Islam with a variety of universal existential questions.

15. This last question is adapted from Griffith and Griffith, *Encountering the Sacred*, 58.

16. Some Christians believe the only legitimate reason to divorce is if one member of the marriage has committed adultery (Matthew 19:9), and some Christian counselors express this view clearly to their clients. While it is unavoidable that we therapists will have opinions about the choices our clients are facing, and while our spiritual perspectives may color some of our opinions, it is an ethical breach to push our opinions on our clients in the way this client reported.

17. Readers familiar with IFS therapy will recognize the approach I am using here.

18. Psalm 13:1.

19. Job 3:11.

Chapter 9

1. Griffith and Griffith, *Encountering the Sacred*, 218.

2. *Moral injury* refers to the damage we do to ourselves by violating our moral values. Much attention is being given to the moral injury suffered by soldiers who have participated in or witnessed acts of inhumanity, but persons in other contexts can wound themselves emotionally, relationally, and spiritually by acting against the grain of conscience and spirit. Syracuse University sponsors a Moral Injury Project, with an excellent website: http://moralinjuryproject.syr.edu/. And Brock and Lettini have written *Soul Repair*, a helpful book addressing moral injury from a spiritual perspective.

3. This pragmatic approach is the one put forth by William James, the founder of the field of psychology of religion. In 1902, in *The Varieties of Religious Experience*, James wrote, "Not its origin, but *the way in which it works on the whole*, is [the] final test of a belief. . . . In the end it had to come to our empiricist criterion:

By their fruits ye shall know them, not by their roots" (emphasis in original).

4. Remember: the word "religion" shares etymology with the word "ligament." Healthy religion connects.

5. Quoted in Shapiro, *Perennial Wisdom*, 53.

6. Galatians 2:20 RSV.

7. I also highly recommend Peterson and Seligman's study of positive character traits in *Character Strengths and Virtues*. One of the great things about their book is that they attempt to look at virtues that are recognized across cultures and are, thus, more universally human.

8. Exodus 20:13.

9. Micah 6:8.

10. This is what Lao Tzu critiqued in Confucianism, what Buddha critiqued in Hinduism, and what the Old Testament prophets and Jesus critiqued in Judaism.

11. James Griffith describes a tragic case where the parents of an eleven-year-old boy, believing he had been healed of insulin-dependent diabetes, allowed him to slip into a coma and die, this with the encouragement of a traveling evangelist and some members of their church (Griffith, *Religion That Heals*, 116; Griffith and Griffith, *Encountering the Sacred*, 215–19).

12. More precisely, Marx called religion "the opium of the people." This phrase is from the introduction to his *A Contribution to the Critique of Hegel's Philosophy of Right*, begun in 1843 but not published until after his death.

13. Another way spirituality and religion become harmful that you may encounter in your clinical practice but that, for reasons of space, I do not discuss in this chapter, is when spirituality and religion interact negatively with a mental illness. Sometimes harmful religion can actually activate a psychiatric illness. We will encounter this later in this chapter in the cases of Rich, whose spiritual injury caused PTSD, and Kelly, whose fear-heavy religion adds to the burden of her mood disorder.

It can happen the other way also. A psychiatric disorder can amplify the negative effect of harmful religion. Depression can darken our relationship with God or our spiritual community, psychosis can wreak havoc on our perceptions of God, and OCD can intensify the impact of guilt-based religion, as it does for Gary, whom you will also meet later in this chapter.

If you're interested in reading more about how mental illness and religion can interact in unhealthy ways, and what to do about that, I'll refer you again to Griffith's *Religion That Heals*.

14. This is the definition offered by Oakley and Kinmond in *Breaking the Silence*. They also note that spiritual abuse can include "manipulation and exploitation, enforced accountability, censorship of decision making, requirements for secrecy and silence, pressure to conform, misuse of scripture or the pulpit to control behaviour, requirement of obedience to the abuser, the suggestion that the abuser has a 'divine' position, and isolation from others, especially those external to the abusive context" (25). Another good treatment of spiritual abuse is a book by Johnson and VanVonderen, *Subtle Power*. They define spiritual abuse as "mistreatment of a person who is in need of help, support or greater spiritual empowerment, with the result of weakening, undermining or decreasing that person's spiritual empowerment" (20). I regret that limitations of space prevent me from giving the concept more attention in this book. I encourage you to read more about it in either of these excellent resources.

15. Griffith, *Religion That Heals*, 97 (emphasis added).

16. All three examples in the preceding paragraph are of men: Buddha, Jesus, Muhammad. While there are certainly female reformers within many of the major religions—Mary Baker Eddy, who founded the Christian Science movement, and Ellen White, who helped establish Seventh Day Adventism—and while Wicca and other Earth religions are often female-led, the history of the dominant religions is inseparable from the history of patriarchy.

17. This is a metaphor Jesus uses. See Matthew 9:14–17, Mark 2:21–22, and Luke 5:33–39.

18. Respect means seeing our clients as persons of value, believing they're doing the best they can applying the survival strategies they currently know in the difficult circumstances in which they find themselves, and trusting that they understand their situation better than we understand it and they'll know better than we do what they need to do about it. Empathy means feeling in ourselves some of what it might feel like to be in their shoes, allowing what we feel to resonate in us, and letting clients see and hear that we're affected by them. Curiosity means restraining our tendency to prejudge and assign people to categories, and seeking, instead, to know more about them and let them teach us.

19. Griffith, *Religion That Heals*, 93. These are slight adaptations of the questions he suggests.

20. Ibid., 175, emphasis added.

21. Most readers will be familiar with problematic texts in Judaism, Christianity, and Islam, but may not be aware of similarly problematic texts in Buddhism and Hinduism. According to Buddhist Scripture, for instance, the Buddha initially refused to receive women into his sangha [religious community], and when he did, he placed eight rules upon them that were not required of men. The Buddhist Scriptures also have teachings that justify slavery, connecting it with beliefs in karma and reincarnation. The Hindu Scriptures include passages that promote sexism and justify slavery. Let it also be noted that, as with the Abrahamic religions, the Scriptures of both these religions also contain passages that oppose sexism and slavery.

22. Ephesians 4:15.

Chapter 10

1. Yogananda, *Second Coming*, 11–16.

2. This one sentence—"We are part of God, and God is part of us"—contains centuries and libraries of spiritual understanding,

misunderstanding, disagreement, and paradox. I mean it in the wonderful way Arthur Osborne puts it in this sentence: "A Realized Man [*sic*] cannot say 'I am God' but can say 'I am not other-than-God'" (Osborne, *Be Still*, 57).

3. You might recall Marie, in chapter 8, saying, "I want a divorce," and my response of mirroring and asking her what else she noticed when she said those words. (See page 123.) The intervention there is informed by the perspective here, that declarations of clarity are often a way God becomes present and active in a human life.

4. There is much more power in "I won't" than in "I can't."

5. The word for this in the Abrahamic traditions is *sin*. In the Eastern religions it is *illusion* and *delusion*. I'll add a more psychological word, *dissociation*, and say this: things fall apart for us, inside and out, because we dissociate from our spiritual selves. The psychological tradition, of course, ascribes psychopathology to biological factors (chemical imbalances), social factors (attachment injuries and trauma), and psychological factors (defenses, fixations, addictions, and neuroses). These understandings are also true, and what I am saying here, from a spiritual perspective, is not incompatible with these bio-psycho-social understandings. But from a spiritual perspective, psychopathology is the adaptation of a self that has dissociated from its connection with Love.

6. "True self" is a phrase used by both psychoanalyst Donald Winnicott and Christian contemplative Thomas Merton. See Winnicott, "Ego Distortion," and Merton, *New Seeds*, 34–35.

7. Winnicott and Merton also both use the phrase "false self."

8. Cozolino, *Neuroscience*.

Chapter 11

1. Bair, *Living from the Heart*, 26.

2. This phrase, used in many circles, is one I first encountered in Sensorimotor Psychotherapy training.

3. I learned this intervention from Griffith and Griffith, *Encountering the Sacred*, and it has become my all-time-favorite way of intervening with clients who believe in God. If you want to know more about this intervention and how to use it, I highly recommend Griffith and Griffith's book.

4. Matthew 14:22–33.

Chapter 12

1. Spiritual countertransference also includes your response to the therapy situation itself: to its limits, to your limits, to the responsibility of your role, to the uncertainty that are near-constants, to the power differential between you and your client, and more. If this were a longer treatment of spiritual countertransference, I would include this aspect in my definition and address it further. But for sake of simplicity and brevity in this chapter, I am limiting myself to the abridged definition I've provided.

2. If, like me, you believe that the entirety of the human experience is spiritual, then, technically, everything your client ever tells you is spiritual, every experience your client has with you is spiritual, and every experience you have as a therapist is an experience of spiritual countertransference. This "everything is spiritual" perspective, of course, is so broad that it dulls the sharp edge of practical utility, and I am doing my best, in this chapter and throughout the book, to be true to my understanding of the spiritual substance of all reality but also to use clinical examples that feel "clearly spiritual."

3. Genia, "Religious Issues"; Miller, *Incorporating Spirituality*; Griffith, "Managing Religious Countertransference"; Hodge, "Using Spiritual Interventions"; and Peteet, "Struggles with God."

4. Griffith, "Managing Religious Countertransference," 197.

5. Psalm 42:7.

6. Understanding spiritual countertransference as a barrier to be overcome aligns with what is called the "classical" understanding. When Freud coined the term "countertransference," he

described it as an unwanted intrusion of issues from the therapist's past into the therapeutic dyad. For Freud, the work of therapy was to make the unconscious conscious through the interpretation of the transference; for the transference to unfold in a way that surfaces the patient's unconscious issues, the therapist must provide a blank slate upon which those issues can be projected with a degree of purity. For therapy to work, the therapist must thus keep the therapy space free of his own unresolved issues that might disturb the theoretically uncontaminated emergence of the transference. (See Freud, "Future Prospects" and "Observations on Transference-Love.")

After Freud, psychotherapy theory soon acknowledged that a real human being cannot be a blank slate, that no therapist is ever so fully actualized that he does not bring his own issues into the therapy space, and that what therapists feel in response to their patients is evoked not merely by the therapist's past experience but by the present experience with this patient. Theorists like Winnicott ("Hate in the Countertransference"), Heimann ("On Countertranference"), and Racker (*Transference and Countertransference*) took this recognition into account and expanded our understanding of countertransference to mean "all that happens" for the therapist, the therapist's total response to the client, and the act of being in a helping relationship with the client. In this "totalist" understanding (see Kernberg, "Notes on Countertransference"), countertransference includes elements transferred from the therapist's past *and* elements evoked in the present by the client. Countertransference is sometimes a barrier to the work of therapy, and the therapist must try to neutralize or minimize it. But it is also sometimes a valuable source of information and empathy, and the therapist can utilize it in service of connection, understanding, and transformation. In more recent years, intersubjectivity theory (see, e.g., Stolorow, Atwood, and Brandchaft, *Intersubjective Perspective*) and relational psychoanalytic theory (see, e.g., Ogden, *Projective Identification*) have continued to explore this more positive understanding of countertransference, and Cooper-White has written an excellent book (*Shared Wisdom*) showing how the totalist understanding is helpful in the work of pastoral care and counseling.

7. Another reason for giving considerable attention to your own experience has to do with therapeutic presence. I am not saying much about therapeutic presence in this book, but in general I mean the therapist's capacity to use her self, the physical-emotional-spiritual energy of her presence, to help the client feel safe, accepted, accompanied, mindful, courageous, free, creative, powerful, and the like. One of the tools for enhancing therapeutic presence (though "tools" is far too mechanical an image for what happens here) is free-floating mindful awareness—of thoughts, feelings, and particularly physical sensations and impulses. This practice heightens and deepens a sense of spaciousness and energy I feel in myself, and I notice that it affects my clients as well.

8. It has not, however, kept me from writing this book in a way that might be spiritually triggering for you. It's one thing to be sensitive to a client's experience, and another to be so sensitive to you, whose job it is to keep your wits about you in the presence of all sorts of spiritual expression.

9. Substitute any other hot-button issue here: the client who is incredibly wealthy, the client who is choosing to have an abortion, the client who is polyamorous, etc.

10. If there's a particular religious or spiritual perspective that is prevalent in your community (for example, biblical literalists, Muslims, Native Americans, and others), it's important to get to know that perspective as deeply as you can. The lives of your clients are likely to be stongly affected, directly or indirectly, by this perspective.

11. "Try letting" is an interesting and wonderful little directive, isn't it? It's got an active component, the word "try," and a receptive component, the word "letting." I think those two words, together like that, convey a lot about the nature of spiritual

experience. Three letters worth of doing, trying, and intention. And seven letters of receiving, allowing, and surrender.

Chapter 13

1. I can recommend this specific opportunity for further learning because I helped develop it: a training program in Spiritually Integrated Psychotherapy that will be offered through ACPE (www.acpe.edu) beginning in 2020. (The program is being piloted in 2019, alongside publication of this book, and will be offered more widely beginning in 2020.) The program includes a thirty-hour continuing education curriculum and case consultation with an approved consultant. It will reinforce many of the strategies described in this book and connect you with highly trained therapists who can support you in growing your skills in this way of working.

Bibliography

Abu-Raiya, H., K. I. Pargament, J. J. Exline, and Q. Agbaria. "Prevalence, Predictors, and Implications of Religious/Spiritual Struggles among Muslims." *Journal for the Scientific Study of Religion* 54 (2015): 631–48.

Abu-Raiya, H., K. I. Pargament, N. Krause, and G. Ironson. "Robust Links between Religious/Spiritual Struggles, Psychological Distress, and Well-Being in a National Sample of American Adults." *American Journal of Orthopsychiatry* 85 (2015): 565–75.

Abu-Raiya, H., K. I. Pargament, A. Weissberger, and J. J. Exline. "An Examination of Religious/Spiritual Struggle among Israeli Jews." *International Journal for the Psychology of Religion* 26 (2016): 61–79.

Bair, Puran. *Living from the Heart: Heart Rhythm Meditation for Energy, Clarity, Peace, Joy, and Inner Power.* New York: Three Rivers Press, 1998.

Balboni, M. J., and T. A. Balboni. *Hostility to Hospitality: Spirituality and Professional Socialization within Medicine.* New York: Oxford University Press, 2019.

Berry, Wendell. "The Peace of Wild Things." In *Collected Poems, 1957–1982*. San Francisco: North Point Press, 1985.

Bourgeault, Cynthia. *The Heart of Centering Prayer: Nondual Christianity in Theory and Practice*. Boulder, CO: Shambhala, 2016.

Brock, Rita Nakashima, and Gabriella Lettini. *Soul Repair: Recovering from Moral Injury after War*. Boston: Beacon Press, 2012.

Chittister, Joan. *Welcome to the Wisdom of the World and Its Meaning for You: Universal Spiritual Insights from Five Religious Traditions*. Grand Rapids: Eerdmans, 2007.

Chodron, Penna. *How to Meditate*. 1997; repr., Boulder, CO: Sounds True.

Cooper-White, Pamela. *Shared Wisdom: Use of the Self in Pastoral Care and Counseling*. Minneapolis: Fortress Press, 2004.

Cozolino, Louis. *The Neuroscience of Human Relationships: Attachment and the Developing Social Brain*. 2nd ed. New York: W. W. Norton, 2014.

Desai, K. M., and K. I. Pargament. "Predictors of Growth and Decline following Spiritual Struggles." *International Journal for the Psychology of Religion* 25 (2015): 42–56.

Finley, James. *Christian Meditation: Experiencing the Presence of God*. New York: Harper Collins, 2004.

Freud, Sigmund. "The Future Prospects of Psycho-Analytic Therapy." In *The Standard Edition of the Complete Psychological Works of Sigmund Freud*. Edited and translated by J. Strachey, 11:141–51. 1910; repr., New York: Norton, 2000.

Freud, Sigmund. "Observations on Transference-Love." In *The Standard Edition of the Complete Psychological Works of Sigmund Freud*. Edited and translated by J. Strachey, 12:157–71. 1915; repr., New York: Norton, 2000.

Genia, V. "Religious Issues in Secularly Based Psychotherapy." *Counseling and Values* 44 (2000): 213–21.

Goleman, Daniel, and Richard J. Davidson. *Altered Traits: Science Reveals How Meditation Changes Your Mind, Brain, and Body*. New York: Penguin Random House, 2017.

Griffith, James L. "Managing Religious Countertransference in Clinical Settings." *Psychiatric Annals* 36 (2006): 196–204.

———. *Religion That Heals, Religion That Harms: A Guide for Clinical Practice.* New York: Guilford Press, 2010.

Griffith, James L., and Melissa Elliott Griffith. *Encountering the Sacred in Psychotherapy: How to Talk with People about Their Spiritual Lives.* New York: Guilford Press, 2002.

Griffiths, Bede. *River of Compassion.* Springfield, IL: Templegate Publications, 1987.

Gubi, Peter Madsen. *Prayer in Counselling and Psychotherapy: Exploring a Hidden Meaningful Dimension.* London: Jessica Kingsley, 2008.

Harris, Dan. *Meditation for Fidgety Skeptics: A 10% Happier How-To Book.* New York: Random House, 2017.

Heimann, P. "On Countertranference." *International Journal of Psychoanalysis* 31 (1950): 81–84.

Helminski, Kabir Edmund. *Living Presence.* New York: Jeremy P. Tarcher/Putnam, 1992.

Hodge, David. "Implicit Spiritual Assessment." *Social Work* 58, no. 3 (2013): 223–30.

———. "Using Spiritual Interventions in Practice: Developing Some Guidelines from Evidence-Based Practice." *Social Work* 56, no. 2 (2011): 149–58.

James, William. *The Varieties of Religious Experience: A Study in Human Nature.* 1902. http://www.gutenberg.org/ebooks/621.

Johanson, Greg, and Ron Kurtz. *Grace Unfolding: Psychotherapy in the Spirit of the Tao-te Ching.* New York: Bell Tower, 1991.

Johnson, David, and Jeff VanVonderen. *The Subtle Power of Spiritual Abuse: Recognizing and Escaping Spiritual Manipulation and False Spiritual Authority within the Church.* Minneapolis: Bethany House Publishers, 2005.

Kabat-Zinn, Jon. *Wherever You Go, There You Are: Mindfulness Meditation in Everyday Life.* New York: Hyperion, 1994.

Kahneman, Daniel. *Thinking, Fast and Slow.* New York: Farrar, Straus and Giroux, 2011.

Keating, Thomas. *Invitation to Love: The Way of Christian Contemplation*. 20th anniv. ed. London: Continuum, 2012.

Kernberg, Otto. "Notes on Countertransference." *Journal of the American Psychoanalytic Association* 13 (1965): 38–56.

Kornfield, Jack. *Meditation for Beginners: Six Guided Meditations for Insight, Inner Clarity, and Cultivating a Compassionate Heart*. Boulder, CO: Sounds True, 2004.

La Torre, Mary Ann. "Prayer in Psychotherapy: An Important Perspective." *Perspectives in Psychiatric Care* 40, no. 1 (2004): 2–40.

Laird, Martin. *Into the Silent Land: A Guide to the Christian Practice of Contemplation*. New York: Oxford University Press, 2006.

Lamott, Anne. *Help, Thanks, Wow: Three Essential Survival Prayers*. New York: Riverhead Books, 2012.

Magaletta, P. R. "Prayer in Psychotherapy: A Model for Its Use, Ethical Considerations, and Guidelines for Practice." *Journal of Psychology and Theology* 26, no. 4 (1998): 322–30.

Maynard, Elizabeth, and Jill Snodgrass, eds. *Understanding Pastoral Counseling*. New York: Springer, 2015.

Mendez, A., and R. Fine. "A Short History of the British School of Object Relations and Ego Psychology." *Bulletin of the Menninger Clinic* 40 (1976): 357–82.

Merton, Thomas. *New Seeds of Contemplation*. New York: New Directions Books, 1961.

Miller, G. *Incorporating Spirituality in Counseling and Psychotherapy: Theory and Technique*. Hoboken, NJ: John Wiley & Sons, 2002.

Mother Teresa. *Come Be My Light: The Private Writings of the Saint of Calcutta*. Edited by Brian Kolodiejchuk. New York: Doubleday, 2007.

Murray, Henry A., and Clyde Kluckhohn. *Personality in Nature, Society, and Culture*. 1948. 2nd ed. New York: Knopf, 1971.

Oakley, Lisa, and Kathryn Kinmond. *Breaking the Silence on Spiritual Abuse*. London: Palgrave Macmillan, 2013.

Ogden, Pat, and Janina Fisher. *Sensorimotor Psychotherapy: Interventions for Trauma and Attachment*. New York: W. W. Norton, 2015.

Ogden, T. H. *Projective Identification and Psychotherapeutic Technique*. Northvale, NJ: Jason Aronson, 1982.

Oliver, Mary. *New and Selected Poems*. Vol. 1. Boston: Beacon Press, 1992.

Orr, Gregory. *Concerning the Book That Is the Body of the Beloved*. Port Townsend, WA: Copper Canyon Press, 2005.

Osborne, Arthur. *Be Still, It Is the Wind That Sings*. Tiruvannamalai, India: Sri Ramanasraman, 2000.

Pargament, Kenneth I. Presentation at AAPCSE Annual Meeting, Kanuga Conference Center, Hendersonville, North Carolina, October 19, 2018.

———. *Spiritually Integrated Psychotherapy: Understanding and Addressing the Sacred*. New York: Guilford Press, 2007.

Peteet, J. R. "Struggles with God: In the Treatment of a Trauma Survivor." *Journal of the American Academy of Psychoanalysis and Dynamic Psychiatry* 37, no. 1 (2009): 165–74.

Peterson, Christopher, and Martin Seligman. *Character Strengths and Virtues: A Handbook and Classification*. Washington, DC: American Psychological Association, 2004.

Pew Research Center. "America's Changing Religious Landscape," May 12, 2015, pewforum.org.

Plante, Thomas G. *Spiritual Practices in Psychotherapy: Thirteen Tools for Enhancing Psychological Health*. Washington, DC: American Psychological Association, 2009.

Porges, Stephen, and Ryan Howes. "Wearing Your Heart on Your Face: The Polyvagal Circuit in the Consulting Room." Psychotherapy Networker, September/October 2013, https://www.psychotherapynetworker.org/magazine/article/160/point-of-view.

Racker, H. *Transference and Countertransference*. New York: International University Press, 1968.

Reninger, Elizabeth. *Meditation Now: A Beginner's Guide*. Berkeley, CA: Althea Press, 2014.

Renzetti, Elizabeth. "Bruce Springsteen on Struggling with Depression, Family and Donald Trump." *Globe and Mail*, October 21, 2016, updated May 17, 2018, theglobeandmail.com.

Richards, P. Scott, and Allen E. Bergin. *A Spiritual Strategy for Counseling and Psychotherapy*. 2nd ed. Washington, DC: American Psychological Association, 2005.

Rizzuto, Ana-María. *Birth of the Living God: A Psychoanalytic Study*. Chicago: University of Chicago Press, 1979.

Rohr, Richard. *Immortal Diamond: The Search for Our True Self*. San Francisco: Jossey-Bass, 2013.

Rossiter-Thornton, John. "Prayer in Psychotherapy." *Alternative Therapies in Health and Medicine* 6, no. 1 (January 2000): 125–28.

Shapiro, Rami. *Perennial Wisdom for the Spiritually Independent*. Woodstock, VT: SkyLight Paths Publishing, 2013.

Smith, Huston. *The World's Religions: Our Great Wisdom Traditions*. 50th anniv. ed. New York: HarperCollins, 2008.

Sperry, Len. *Spirituality in Clinical Practice: Theory and Practice of Spiritually Oriented Psychotherapy*. 2nd ed. New York: Routledge, 2012.

Stolorow, R., G. E. Atwood, and B. Brandchaft. *The Intersubjective Perspective*. Northvale, NJ: Jason Aronson, 1994.

Taft, Michael W. *The Mindful Geek: Secular Meditation for Smart Skeptics*. Oakland, CA: Cephalopod Rex, 2015.

Thich Nhat Hanh. *The Miracle of Mindfulness: An Introduction to the Practice of Meditation*. Boston: Beacon Press, 1975.

———. *Peace Is Every Step: The Path of Mindfulness in Everyday Life*. New York: Bantam Books, 1991.

Vieten, Cassandra, and Shelley Scammell. *Spiritual and Religious Competencies in Clinical Practice: Guidelines for Psychotherapists and Mental Health Professionals*. Oakland, CA: New Harbinger, 2015.

Way of Chuang Tzu. Translated by Thomas Merton. London: Burns & Oakes, 1995.

Welwood, John. *Toward a Psychology of Awakening: Buddhism, Psychotherapy, and the Path of Personal and Spiritual Transformation.* Boston: Shambhala, 2002.

Williams, Mark, and Danny Penman. *Mindfulness: A Practical Guide to Finding Peace in a Frantic World.* London: Piatkus, 2014.

Winnicott, Donald W. "Ego Distortion in Terms of True and False Self." In Winnicott, *The Maturational Processes and the Facilitating Environment: Studies in the Theory of Emotional Development,* 140–52. Madison, CT: International Universities Press, 1994 (1960/1965).

———. "Hate in the Countertransference." In Winnicott, *Collected Papers: Through Paediatrics to Psycho-Analysis,* 194–203. New York: Brunner/Mazel, 1992 (1949).

———. "The Location of Cultural Experience" In Winnicott, *Playing & Reality.* 1971; repr., New York: Routledge, 1991.

Yogananda, Paramahansa. *The Second Coming of Christ: The Resurrection of the Christ within You: A Revelatory Commentary on the Original Teachings of Jesus.* 2004; repr., Los Angeles: Self-Realization Fellowship, 2015.

Index